A'Weighted:

A Journey between The *Weight* & The *Wait*

Juanita D. Jones

Dedication

To the Great Almighty God because without Him I am Nothing! All praise and credit goes to Him for anything that's accomplished in my life. I was born, designed, and purposed to WIN and to fulfill my purpose for HIS will. He is and always will be the REASON.

To my best friend, the peas to my carrots, my amazing husband Steve. Thank you for being my #1 supporter. I'm so grateful to live this life with you. You have loved and accepted me literally and figuratively through the "thick" and the "not so thick". I love you to Life!

My sons Jalil and Jalen... You are the two main reasons that I don't give up, keep believing, and keep dreaming. Thank you Jalil for reminding me when I was so "calorie conscious" and unable to enjoy the simple things in life to just "LIVE". Your reminder awakened me from a trance, and I'm thankful for God using you as an instrument

to speak to me! Jalen, thank you for loving
me no matter how big or small I became.
Your genuine care and concern is noticed
and it melts my heart. I love you both more
than you'll ever know!

To my phenomenal sister 'Vee'… I will and
have always been forever grateful for you.
"Me" love you to pieces! (Insider) ;).

Last but certainly not least, to all the people
that have battled, are battling, or in pursuit to
battle the "weight" journey… There's only
one you and they'll never be another. You
are destined to be the absolute BEST that
you can be and there is nothing on this earth
that can stop you from achieving it! This
one's written for YOU!

Acknowledgements

I give honor my pastors who selflessly pour into me, my family and thousands of lives week in and week out: Bishop George L. & Pastor April R. Davis of Impact Church Jacksonville. There are simply not enough words of gratitude that I could express for you teaching, living, and demonstrating the word of God on a daily basis. I love you both immensely!

Angelica Echevarria, for your patience and for using your amazing God-given photography skills to do my photo shoots. I am tremendously blessed to have worked with you on several projects, and I thank you.

Thank you to the awesome Fiverr and Amazon Publishing teams for providing excellent and fast services when it came to editing, formatting, creative art, and publishing.

To my husband Steve, thank you for lending me your eyeballs to read and ears to listen to me vent on a day to day basis. Thanks for letting me cry on days I felt like a blubbering mess, but nevertheless you loved me just the same.

Fatima Kargbo – My 'bff" - There is simply not enough 'thank you's' in the universe that I could ever give you for being such a true friend. I've said it before and I'll continue to say it – you are a God send and I love you dearly.

Last, but certainly far from least, to all the people that made me feel inferior, not good enough, who criticized me, ridiculed me, gossiped about me, passed over me, stolen and cheated me, and for the ones that made me feel 'small', despite your words and/or actions, I'M. STILL. HERE. I'm better, wiser, more matured, and stronger because of you. Thank you for being an instrument in helping quicken my metamorphosis from a caterpillar into a butterfly.

Foreword

I started writing this book in the summer of 2016, because I felt the pressure of having to do a sophomore book release after finishing my first book The Frustrated Dreamer (TFD). Also because I'm such a strong type 'A' personality, I believed it had to be done and it had to be done right away. I went through the motions - storyline structure, cover photos, scribble pads, etc., the same processes I went through when I wrote TFD (which was written, edited, proofread, and self-published all in only 6 months' time - an incredible feat for a first time author). I quickly learned that the process for this book certainly wouldn't be the same case.

On July 26th 2016, I took a massive leap of faith without a safety net and left my corporate job to dive headfirst into my business, Edible Blessings, LLC (Custom Cakes & Desserts) - a love I have been having an affair with since winter 2002 part time while I continued to work a full time job. For almost 16 years, I worked double duty - 40 hours on my "9-5" for various corporate companies, then would come home and work another 20-40 hours for myself. So after finishing TFD, God gave me the title and the subject for what you're about to read.

"Lord, No way! I've got way too much on my plate with being a mom, wife, volunteer and with running Edible Blessings to start writing another book! I finally just started working full time with my own business (which is a monster of a transition and incredibly scary), and I simply don't have time to write yet another book!" Have you ever felt like you were talking to a brick wall? That's what God made me feel like when I made up the quick rebuttal, knowing good and well that I can't run from my purpose.

There are much deeper, intertwined, diseased, and rotting roots attached to 'A'weighted'. Issues that seem to run perpetually deep and are still being untangled as you read this foreword. I have started and stopped the process of writing more times than I can count. Why? Simply because the thought of having to be THIS vocal and transparent in an area that has haunted me since I was a young girl caused me detriment. It meant that I had to face demons, come to some real conclusions, and ultimately look at myself naked in the mirror both (figuratively and literally), and deal with the iniquities head on. I wasn't ready for it.

One thing I said I'd never do was write something that was a bunch of bull. It's not in my character to be anything other than *real*. No one wants to read or hear a bunch of fluff from a "perfect" person who has no problems and the world is made of marshmallows and gumdrops. Yeah, right! I'm far from having it all together; as a matter of fact I've got a whole lot of spilled mess that needs to be wiped away.

I've realized that I'm not alone, and that so many other people (men as well as women) deal with the exact same inhibitions but pretend that everything is peaches and cream when it's really liver and onions (sorry for those who actually like liver, but you get the analogy). I've recognized that my putting off getting this book done was because I subconsciously was waiting for myself to finally have a story of "victory" in this area to be able to share with you, so that you in turn could have a living witness that could say, "Hey I've got it all figured out and I've got it altogether ". Baloney!

I've come to the conclusion even after writing TFD that you never truly "arrive". Growth & Evolvement? Yes. But arrive? No. I completed that chapter in my life, and afterwards there were still MANY more days that lied ahead when I was frustrated, busted and disgusted. I recognized that the timing for when it was written and released was not only a blessing to those who have read or listened to it, but it was actually written as my own self manual for things I would encounter in the days, weeks and even years following its release. God's truly got a sense of humor and is no doubt the MASTER orchestrator. I'm choosing to follow his lead, because he's never led me anywhere I didn't need to go for the sake of purpose. So it is written - my journey "a weights" you.

My Long "A-WEIGHTED" Victory

(Excerpt from The Frustrated Dreamer: When your Dreams are Bigger than your Now)

I can recall a pivotal point in my life when I desired to lose weight to conquer haunting issues with low self-esteem, and more importantly for my health and longevity. I battled with a warped self-image for as long as I can recall and it was deeply rooted. Adding to adolescent issues was the constant "in your face" reminders of video vixens, magazine ads, TV commercials, and other propaganda where the women depicted as 'beautiful' looked nothing like me.

As an adult my self-perception worsened to the point that the enemy had me thinking that not only would I never lose the weight, but I was actually convinced that I *couldn't* lose the weight! I believed that it was impossible, so I acted accordingly by doing absolutely nothing to change it. To add insult to injury, I gave birth to my two beautiful sons who I wouldn't trade for the world, but the pregnancies wrecked even more havoc on my body image and self-esteem.

I thank God for my wonderful husband who always told me there was nothing wrong with me and I was beautiful to him. But, he could have told me a million times and it still wouldn't have mattered because I was mentally defeated. So what became the final straw? What was my breaking point? How did I finally defeat the lies of the enemy?

In the spring of 2013, I went to Daytona Beach, FL with my family to celebrate my birthday which happened to during spring break time for college students. We were having a great time, until we decided to visit the boardwalk. As we walked along the arcades and the other typical boardwalk attractions, everything seemed to stand still in my head. There I was, staring at my reflection in the glass of a pizza shop, while a herd of young, tight, firm bodied young women pranced by me.

Without even realizing it, tears started rolling down my face. I was so disappointed and unhappy with myself and I hated the reflection looking back at me. Sadly, all I could think about was "I really just want to eat a slice of pizza". The pizza would comfort me from feeling the pain and the misery of being trapped in a body I really hated. Eat it now, and regret it seconds later was the story of my life.

My family had no idea that I was so upset at a time that was supposed to be enjoyed. I dried my tears and hid my feelings for the remainder of the trip for their sake, but that short moment staring at the reflection in the pizza shop window was branded in my head forever. I had seen my reflection a thousand times before, but it was something different about seeing it in a setting where I felt like a whale out of water (literally) surrounded by a bunch of 'mermaids'.

I went through all the same old lies, which I later realized were actually excuses – "I can't lose weight", "it's too hard", "it will be a waste of my time", etc. Frustration was an understatement! I tried all the dumb gimmicks on the market for a quick fix, and would start and stop exercise regimes more times than there are days in a year and failed every time. I had no will power and no drive until finally I received a revelation that I was good enough in the eyes of God just where I was at that point. I was qualified to do whatever I put my mind to do, and I kept reciting that I could do all things through Christ who gives me strength! [1]

With the help of the Lord through prayer and meditation, as well receiving the encouragement from a good friend (she knows who she is), my warped perception was finally broken! I got serious about changing my life by applying basic, common sense practices.

I immediately (and *immediately* is the key word!) changed my eating habits and began a rigorous exercise regime. Waiting until the next week or the next month wasn't an option. I made my goals attainable by making them small, rather than setting a grandiose goal that would be close to impossible to keeping. I solicited the support of complete strangers who were on the same journey that wouldn't pass judgment, but would offer sound advice and encouragement.

I would be lying if I said it was easy, because it was everything but that, but I kept going! One day at a time, one meal at a time, one workout at a time, one prayer at a time. I did as much as I could, and when I could with no excuses. If I missed a workout, I made it up. If I ate something that wasn't considered healthy, I made up for it by flushing out my body and going extra hard. I didn't deprive myself, and I certainly didn't use the "D" word –Diet (more on this later)!   I made a *lifestyle change*, not a quick temporary fix through gimmicks and diet fads.

---

[1] Philippians 4:13. 2015. New Living Translation Holy Bible.

After 1 year and a swimming pool full of sweat and tears later, I conquered what the enemy held over my head all of my life (oh so I thought)! It might not seem like such a huge feat to someone else, but for me it was a complete renewing of my mind, body, self-esteem, and my life!

I was led to use my own ups and downs, my own successes and setbacks to be a learning opportunity for those of you who have dealt with or currently dealing with the same hurdles regarding body image, self-esteem, and having the ability and stamina to make the necessary changes. Change is never easy. It comes with a great deal of discomfort and forces you to look yourself in the face and deal with cold hard facts that most likely have been avoided.

My prayer is that as you absorb this information, that you take what you receive and apply it as it fits to your needs and lifestyle. There is no "one size fits all" approach to becoming a healthier and better 'you', but there are practical, common sense steps that can be implemented to launch you into the right direction.

The following are the top 10 lessons I learned on my own weight journey that I continue to apply today:

1. ***If you really want to change your life then you MUST change every aspect of it.*** Don't half step on anything. Give it all or nothing! Even if your all starts out being only 50%, its more than if you give it nothing.
2. ***The key to change is having an agenda.*** You must have a plan in place and WRITE IT DOWN! What you don't see, you easily forget

and fall back into old habits. For example, if you are in pursuit of losing weight, it's a good idea to start writing down what you eat on a daily basis for a short season. Why is that important? If you don't write down what you've eaten for the day, you can easily consume way more than you planned because you unconsciously indulge.

3. ***Set small, attainable goals.*** Write down what you want to do and an estimated timeframe on when you want to achieve them. Mark off one goal at a time as they are reached and celebrate each milestone.

4. ***Be accountable!*** Have someone you trust help you be accountable to stick with your goals. They will be there to give you a kick in the behind when you need it most to stay on track. NO EXCUSES!

5. ***Split your life into work and play time, and have a balance.*** Tipping the scale too far in one direction or the other can be disastrous. Your work time is what you absolutely *have* to do (going to work, paying bills, going to school, etc.), while your play time is what you have a choice to do (play video games, social media, watching TV, etc.).

6. ***Consider your habits and routines of daily life.*** To radically change anything in your life you should ideally change your environment. In my case, I had to change the food I was buying and eating, and the amount of exercise I was doing to see a change in my body. I even had to start watching the places I would go because there could be possible

food temptations that would entice me to get off track.

7. ***Put a value on your time because whether you believe it or not, your time is valuable!*** It's the one thing you can't get back once it's gone and you can't buy more of it. Use it wisely!

8. ***Everyday wasted doing nothing is a day closer to you getting nothing!*** Everyday used to obtain a dream is a day closer to a dream manifested. If your dream is to be the best 'you' that you can be, then it's going to take YOU to achieve it!

9. ***It's Ok to be Human.*** You are not perfect and won't hit the nail on the head every single time. Learn to give yourself some slack and learn to forgive yourself! Satan has a way of constantly bringing up past failures, insecurities, disappointments, etc. in order to keep you shackled. Learn from your mistakes, pick yourself up, brush off the dust and just keep going!

10. ***Enjoy the Journey***. Nothing happens overnight and there is always going to be a process. There will be days when you will not feel like doing anything, and days when you will have to just flat out encourage yourself! The key is one day at a time, and one step at a time until one day you look up and your goal is accomplished.

It is my hope that you find comfort in knowing that you are not alone, and you too can accomplish anything you set your mind to achieve. Life is not always going to be a bed of thorn-less roses, but how you react to what life throws your way will either make or break you.

You can either choose to let your current circumstances defeat you, or you can choose to be tired of being tired and change your situation! You were created with a purpose, designed to dominate, and born to win! The best 'you' that you've been waiting for is literally right around the corner. It's time for you to *live* and enjoy life and stop just 'existing'! Let the Journey Begin…

Contents

<u>Disclaimer</u>

The information in this book is not to be used as a diagnosis for any health condition(s). Any information read and implemented is at your own risk. It is highly recommended before starting any lifestyle change that you consult with your primary physician, dietician, and/or certified fitness trainer.The information provided is based on <u>my own personal experiences, research, and solicited expert advice</u>. I am *not* an expert, but I am an expert at my own body, journey, hurdles, and the steps I had to face in order to overcome each hurdle.

It's my prayer that by reading this book that you will find comfort in knowing you are not alone and there is hope! If you see yourself in anything that you read, you now have a platform to help you become the best 'you' possible!

Here's health and happiness on your journey!

\- J

Chapter 1:
The Three D's

*"I tell you the truth, you can say to this **mountain**, 'May you be lifted up and thrown into the sea, and it will happen. But you must really believe it will happen and have no doubt in your heart."* Mark 11:23 NLT[2]

Wait
verb \\\'wāt[3]

- to stay in a place until an expected event happens, until someone arrives, until it is your turn to do something, etc.
- to not do something until something else happens
- to remain in a state in which you expect or hope that something will happen soon

---

[2] Mark 11:23 New Living Translation, Holy Bible
[3] Merriam-Webster Learners Dictionary. 2016. "Wait". http://www.merriam-webster.com/dictionary/wait

Weight

noun \ˈwāt\[4]

- to stay in a place until an expected event happens, until someone arrives, until it is your turn to do something, etc.
- to not do something until something else happens
- to remain in a state in which you expect or hope that something will happen soon

It's a guarantee that in this life, it is inevitable that both waiting and dealing with the weight of anything (our bodies included) will happen. We wait in line at the grocery store, wait in line at an amusement park, and we wait in rush hour traffic. We carry the weight of our careers, the weight of carrying a child on our backs or hips, the weight that shows on a scale. We have no other choice but to wait, but it's the reaction we give in the process of waiting that determines our fate.

Americans spend about **_37 billion hours_** each year waiting. People from all nationalities generally spend approximately six months of their lives waiting in line. That equals about three days a year of queuing

---

[4] Merriam-Webster Learners Dictionary. 2016. "Weight". http://www.merriam-webster.com/dictionary/weight

up.[5] No wonder so many people become impatient with the waiting process and choose to try what is perceived to be a quicker route to their destination. Losing weight is no different. We are often drawn to run to the front of the line through trying the quickest, easiest, and least expensive methods to gain the "perfect" body, only to be left with sheer disappointment. The end result for many is going right back to where we don't want to be: at the back of the line to wait yet again to reach destination "Thin" or destination "Healthy". Who enjoys going back to 'Start'? More than likely the answer is no one!

Waiting doesn't feel good. It isn't satisfying and there is no instant gratification. However, through the process of waiting, we learn to discipline our flesh and the necessary lessons and skills along the way that we would completely miss by skipping the process. Think about it – food cooked in an oven generally tastes much better than food cooked in a microwave. Yes, the microwave is a lot faster than an oven, but the overall quality of the product is vastly different. The slower process of cooking in an oven allows the product to be cooked to perfection, rather than speed up the process being left with a half cooked or over cooked product. Some things are simply worth the wait!

---

[5] Reference.com. 2016. *"How Much Time do we Spend Waiting?"* *https://www.reference.com/science/much-time-spend-waiting-lifetime-2b089985e5384e65?qo=contentSimilarQuestions#*

There are times when waiting, especially when you desperately want something so badly, can feel unbearable. Have you ever had any issues in your life that seemed so gargantuan that they felt impossible to defeat? Problems that felt never-ending? Problems the size of a mountain, compared to you being the size of an ant? If there are three mountains that I have had to faced on a constant basis, nothing sticks out more than the ferocious climbs I endured (and some still enduring) to get over - **Dysmorphia, Diet, and Depression.**

The funny thing about life is the majority of the mountains we face are created from our own imagination. The mind is a powerful contraption. It controls our ways of thinking, our body functions, our emotions, and everything that makes us human. We have the ability to control every thought that's unpleasant from entering and camping out in our minds that would mold and shape our world. Good or bad, the thoughts we entertain will either lead us in a positive direction or down a path of destruction. The thoughts we receive are based on our daily environment and the stimuli we're exposed to on a regular basis. Being surrounded by images that looked nothing like my reflection morphed my thoughts into believing that if I didn't look like "them", then something was wrong with me.

Dysmorphia, Diet and Depression were my mental "Mt. Everest's" that just like the real mountain, required me to endure some of the most treacherous terrains and conditions that I've ever had to experience. It has been a brutal, unapologetic quest. For every step I took, I encountered a new adversity, a new unpleasant discovery, and really discovered what I was collectively made of as a person.

There have been countless days of exhaustion, deliriousness, weariness, torment, and ultimately, the sense of wanting to throw in the towel at every corner. But despite all of the trials and tribulations, I've come to the conclusion that all three mountains must surrender and move out of my way! I've realized it was my mind that made them way bigger and I subconsciously gave them way too much power and authority.

The minute I demanded and stood on my demands that they had to move, every step towards the top became easier but it didn't happen overnight. The largest of the three D's that put me through the most torture (and still from time to time pursues to haunt my thoughts) is that unmerciful 'Mt. Dysmorphia'.

DYSMORPHIA

So there I was on my thirty-something birthday weekend, staring in the window of that pizza shop looking at my reflection staring back at me, and I felt like I was looking in one of those distorted carnival mirrors. Through my watery eyes as I gradually salted my cheeks with tear stains, I believed I looked like the Goodyear blimp, and felt like the Titanic. There was nothing anyone could say to convince me otherwise.

I felt ugly, unattractive, unworthy, blubbery, nasty, sloppy, and the list of negative adjectives that I used to describe myself went on and on. What I was feeling and fighting is what I later discovered as a taboo as something that millions of people secretly deal with that's as common as sliced bread.

I remember saying to myself every morning before my day began, "Shhhh! don't tell anyone that you secretly hate yourself. That you really don't have it all together and that you secretly wish you could look like someone else every waking minute of the day. Don't tell anyone that you hate the reflection staring back at you, and that you walk around day in and day out wearing a mask. Make sure you tuck in those mask strings so no one can see the real you by accident. Oh, and be sure that you don't let anyone know that you always compare your beauty and worth against every other beautiful woman, and always feel inferior and insecure. Last, definitely don't let anyone know that you don't love yourself, and all you see is every flaw that's wrong with you and you often think about taking your own life. Now let's go out into the world with our "happy" mask on and pretend like never before!"

Amazing isn't it? You can work, go to school, go to church, or walk by someone who's a total stranger and have no idea what it's really like to walk in their shoes. I felt like I was the only person in the world that had self-hate and a morphed sense of perception, but I wasn't.

Body Dysmorphic Disorder (also known as BDD and simply as Dysmorphia), is a mental disorder in which a person is "preoccupied with an imagined physical defect or a minor defect that others often cannot see"[6]. Ultimately, people with this disorder see themselves as "ugly" and "unattractive" and often avoid social exposure, seek after plastic surgery try to improve their appearance, or work incredibly hard to hide the perceived defect. Although I am a social and extroverted person, I worked *very* hard with covering what I thought were very noticeable flaws. BDD turns your mind into a prison – exactly what Satan sets out to accomplish. No matter how many affirmations I received from others, I could never see what they saw, and was never happy with accepting myself the way I was created.

Some things I learned while battling the BDD Mountain is that it shares some features of eating disorders such as Anorexia Nervosa and

---

[6]   Body   Dysmorphic   Disorder.   Web   MD   2016. http://www.webmd.com/mental-health/mental-health-body-dysmorphic-disorder

Bulimia. However, the difference is a person with an eating disorder typically worries about weight and the shape of their body, while a person with BDD is more fixated about a specific body part. Sadly, I had symptoms of all three disorders. I went from focusing on the number on the scale and the shape of my body > to not looking at the scale at all out of fear of what it would say but still focused on my shape > to becoming overly obsessed with one particular part of my body.

It is extremely common for people dealing with BDD to take on ritualistic behaviors, such as constantly looking in a mirror, constantly fixing their clothes, fixing their hair, picking at their skin, etc. It is a real disorder that most people don't even recognize or too ashamed and embarrassed to be transparent enough to ask for help. It's also not bias, as it affects both men and women equally, and typically starts during the teen years, aka puberty.

For many years, I secretly dealt with the symptoms of BDD without ever telling anyone out of fear of rejection, embarrassment, being gossiped about, and laughed at by others. That day staring at the pizza shop window made me realize that I was either going to continue to be in mental prison, or I was going to muster up the strength to move the mountain out of the way and do something to change the situation. After years of denial, I started with educating and being brutally honest with myself for the first time ever, and it was liberating.

I wish I could say that I took a magic pill and everything was fixed overnight but it wasn't. I am still a work in progress. It's because of my strong relationship with God and my faith in Him that I was able to dig my way out of the never-ending pit of despair. While I exercised the spiritual, I also had to implement the same in the natural. Some of the signs and symptoms I learned about regarding BDD[7] included but are not limited to the following:

- Being extremely preoccupied with a perceived flaw in appearance that others can't see or appears minor.

- Strong belief that you have a defect in your appearance that makes you deformed or ugly.

- Belief that others take special notice of your appearance in a negative way or mock you (***this is why it is incredibly important to not make fun of someone. You have no idea how much of a negative impact it can have on a person). I was (and still to this day) have been made fun of because of my height.

---

[7] Body Dysmorphic Disorder. Written by Mayo Clinic Staff. Mayo Clinic 2016. http://www.mayoclinic.org/diseases-conditions/body-dysmorphic-disorder/symptoms-causes/dxc-20200938

- Engaging in behaviors aimed at fixing or hiding the perceived flaw that are difficult to resist or control, such as frequently checking the mirror, grooming, etc.

- Attempting to hide flaws with styling, makeup or clothes.

- Constantly comparing your appearance with others.
- Ridiculing the appearance of others to make yourself feel better about your own appearance.

- Always needing reassurance about your appearance from others.

- Having perfectionist tendencies (I battle with this one constantly).

- Seeking frequent cosmetic procedures with little satisfaction (plastic surgery).

- Avoiding social situations.

- Being so preoccupied with appearance that it causes major distress or problems in your social life, work, school or other areas of functioning.

This is by far not a comprehensive list and not all of the above symptoms applied to me, but I had enough to recognize that there was a serious problem that needed to be addressed. I was able to acknowledge and deal with the issues by facing them head on and by fighting them through prayer and exercising wisdom. I realized that what triggered this mountain in my life like most mental disorders stemmed back to me being teased as a child for being "chubby", and later as a teenage into adulthood for being "short". What everyone else thought was cute or funny eventually chipped away at my self-esteem and mental health that stayed with me well into my adult years. I felt robbed of time that I could have been enjoying my life instead of being afflicted.

BDD in a traditional sense usually doesn't get better on its own, and if continuously ignored, it may get worse over time and lead to severe depression, anxiety and may lead to suicidal thoughts – all three of which I have battled. By Faith, I claim total freedom from BDD, although I constantly deal with the residue that's been left behind.
It takes time to retrain the brain from something that's been morphed into it for years. If you need to seek professional guidance, please don't be ashamed or embarrassed to ask for the help.

DIET

Let's face it; this is one of the most hated words in the English dictionary. The minute the word is used, it automatically translates in to other correlated words in our brain such as "restriction", "misery", "boring", "nasty", or even "dreadful". If you're anything like me, you've seen and heard (and probably tried) every diet gimmick on the market –

- The Military diet
- The Green Smoothie diet
- The Grapefruit diet
- The Meal Replacement Shake diet
- The Gluten Free diet
- The No Carb diet
- The Boiled Egg Diet
- The Cabbage Soup diet
- The Apple Cider & Vinegar diet
- The Low Fat diet
- The No Fat diet
- The Green Tea diet
- The Saran Wrap® yourself like a Hoagie Diet
- The Eliminate anything Delicious diet
- The Eat nothing but Air diet
- The Eat like a Rabbit diet…

…And the list of diets, fads and gimmicks goes on until the end of time. As you read down the list, they probably started sounding sillier by the second. Believe me, I have been there and tried all of the popular ones, and even the close to insane ones, and the one conclusion I came to and discovered that research and science has confirmed is that DIETS

SIMPLY DO NOT WORK! It's not even a matter of science, but a matter of common sense that simply can't be stressed enough.

Anything that highly restricts you from eating or drinking anything in its entirety for a period of time in effort to lose a vast amount of weight quickly, is bound to eventually fail. Yes, you will get results and instant gratification, but I know for a fact that the results are temporary because there are no lessons learned along the way. The only proven effective way (through my own experience and from education) to lose weight and keep it off is to change your way of thinking in relation to food, exercise, and how to live a balanced lifestyle.

It goes a bit further then just diet gimmicks. Think about all of the 'diet' foods and drinks on the market. In almost every case, there contents are actually WORSE than eating the full fat or full sugar version of the product. You get suckered into believing that just because the words 'diet', 'fat free' 'carb free' or 'sugar free' is on the label, you're 'home free' to consume as much as humanly possible. This is far from the truth!

According to the Center for Disease Control (CDC) in 2015, More than one-third (34.9% or 78.6 million) of U.S. adults are obese.[8]

---

[8] Adult Obesity Facts. 2015. Center for Disease Control & Prevention. http://www.cdc.gov/obesity/data/adult.html

Understand that the diet industry knows the facts, and it also knows that these facts equal dollar signs. Most reputable nutritionists agree that most diets aren't worth the paper they're printed on and waste both time and money. The real key to losing and keeping weight off is a sound, sustainable eating plan and exercise regime, and then <u>sticking with it</u>, rather than opting for some quick "lose 10 lbs. in 5 days fix". Let's get real: when you *lose* something, you typically have the ability to find it again. If your goal is to not just "lose weight" but to forever "get rid of it", then it takes real discipline, determination, and patience to get real lasting results.

Let's take a look at some of the *real* reasons diets simply aren't effective:

1. ***Diets are temporary.***

The problem with virtually all diets is they require only a short-term mindset. Most people believe diets are all-or-nothing, and rather than making small incremental changes in their lifestyle for permanent results, diets require you to flip your life inside out for a few days or weeks. The issue is once those few days or weeks are over and you return to your old habits (old ways of eating, thinking, etc.), guess what happens? Your body returns to its "normal" state, and in many cases, it doesn't return without extra "friends" - MORE POUNDS.

Most dieters can change eating habits for a week or two (and sometimes a little longer), but most often, the diet only focuses on external changes - "don't eat this, don't eat that." "Drink this and don't drink that". Changing the type of food alone does not create long lasting change, because it doesn't touch on deeply rooted behaviors or patterns that affect the food choices we make in the first place.

Do you eat when you're bored? Scared? Upset? Do you associate food with comfort and security from your childhood or substantial event in your life? I realized I associated food as a way to deal with boredom, and also filled a void for when I was lonely. Food is a just as much a drug as any other addiction. It looks good, smells good, tastes good, and feels good to the soul when being consumed. Just like any other abused drug, if used inappropriately it can be a damaging menace.

Not recognizing the "why" we eat the way we eat, when we eat, or how we eat leads to nowhere other than a vicious cycle of frustration. You lose weight, and then gain it right back and then some. In order to make sustainable changes, you need to explore *why* and *how* we eat.

It's important to understand that it's the small, consistent changes last and big, sudden ones don't. Saying that you'll change everything all at once by plunging head first into a temporary fix with no form of changing your thinking and your relationship with food doesn't change your underlying behavior patterns. It's the slow, steady route that ultimately leads to success.

2. *Diets zap your energy.*

A major problem with diets is that so many of them are extremely low in calories that leave you with very little energy to do your workouts or accomplish everything else. It's possible that you may drop a few pounds in the interim (mostly water weight like in my case), but you'll neglect muscle, resulting in a metabolic downshift that will take you back to square one[9]. This is especially true if you're following one of the ultra-low-carb or no-carb diets.

Carbohydrates are the main energy source for physical activity, and years of research has shown that low-carb diets don't properly support strenuous physical for extended periods of time. Eliminating or drastically reducing any certain form of food (including healthy fats such as avocado, olive oil, and nuts – yes there are GOOD fats and our body

---

[9] The Institute for the Psychology of Eating. 2016. *"3 Reasons Why Diets Don't Work." http://psychologyofeating.com/3-reasons-diets-dont-work/*

needs it!), can cause adverse effects with your goal to shed weight. Balance is the key.

3. *Diets Suck!*

There's no other way to eloquently put it: dieting just plain sucks!   No one really enjoys being restricted with one of the most pleasurable things on the planet: Food!   All diets have an element of deprivation, and there's often a "do not eat/drink" list of foods to be avoided to be successful. Being so restrictive makes it extremely tough to stick with and enjoy the process of becoming healthier. There's no joy involved in the process, and ultimately most people typically throw in the towel well before they see any results. The stress from so many restrictions causes a rise in cortisol (a hormone) and adrenalin in our bodies, which reduces the ability to burn calories[10], and the exact conditions that makes losing weight a challenge.

You're probably wondering what in the world is "cortisol"? The short answer is it's "a steroid hormone that's made in the adrenal glands."[11]. Most cells in the

---

[10] The Institute for the Psychology of Eating. 2016. *"3 Reasons Why Diets Don't Work." http://psychologyofeating.com/3-reasons-diets-dont-work/*

[11] The Hormone Health Network. 2017. *"What Does Cortisol Do?"* http://www.hormone.org/hormones-and-health/what-do-hormones-do/cortisol

body have cortisol receptors, it affects many different functions in the body. Cortisol can help <u>regulate metabolism</u>, control blood sugar levels, help reduce inflammation and assist with memory. In women, cortisol also supports the developing fetus during pregnancy. These functions make cortisol a crucial hormone to protect overall health.

Think about it – how many times have you started a diet then stopped? If you actually stuck to the diet, did you really enjoy it? Elimination and deprivation is a sure fire way to trigger over indulgence when you finally eat or drink what you've been craving, and can spiral very quickly out of control.

4. *Diets don't address the REAL problem.*
"Why am I fat? I'm not eating fried foods, I'm staying away from desserts and sodas, and I hardly eat all day…but I can't seem to lose a single pound!" That's the question I asked myself over and over again during my weight struggle for years. So why was I still fat (or perceived to be) after all the changes I worked so hard to implement? Fad diets make you believe that you're fat because you're eating too much or not exercising enough, which may be true to an extent, but it's not the full answer to the problem. The truth is that exercise controls only about 20% of your body composition, not the perceived 80% that most people believe.[12] So guess what actually

---

[12] Geary, Kevin. 2016. Rebooted Body 2016. "Why Diets Don't Work". http://rebootedbody.com/why-diets-dont-work/

controls the 80%? You guessed it: FOOD. The formula for losing and keeping the weight off is a full blown lifestyle change that typically includes around 80% nutrition, and 20% exercise.

If you are struggling or have always battled with yo-yo weight (you go back and forth losing and gaining), then more than likely, it's because your metabolism is way out of line. Metabolism is the process by which your body converts what you eat and drink into energy. During this process, calories in food and drinks are combined with oxygen to release the energy your body needs to function.[13]

Several factors determine your individual metabolic rate, including:

- **Your body size and composition.** The bodies of larger people or people who have more muscle typically burn more calories, even as they sleep. You'll learn all about body types in a later chapter.
- **Your sex.** Men usually have less body fat and more muscle than women of the same age and weight, resulting in them burning more calories.
- **Your age.** As you get older, the amount of muscle tends to decrease and fat accounts for more of your weight, slowing down calorie burning. Fight this by getting and staying active!

---

[13] Mayo Clinic Staff. 2016. "Metabolism & Weight Loss: How you burn Calories". http://www.mayoclinic.org/healthy-lifestyle/weight-loss/in-depth/metabolism/art-20046508

Your metabolism may not be functioning properly not because of how little you work out or how much you eat, but because of *what* you eat! Your body is only able to use the food you feed it to fuel it, and if you're not feeding it the right types of foods, then you will literally see the results, aka weight gain.

It's also the same if you eat too little food – your body goes into starvation mode (even if you are considered overweight or obese, you can *still* be starving your body and cause malnourishment). This problem has been one of my biggest issues! I would go all day working and forget to eat or eat very little. I quickly learned that my body stores more fat and that I had done so much damage that my fat cells lost the ability to release the fat that was stored. The good news is that this cycle can be stopped and the damage can be reversed. Learning how to eat properly by changing the way foods are prepared and cooked, as well as the types of foods, and how often certain foods are being consumed is the long term key to successful weight loss.

How do you learn to fully enjoy your life without being monopolized by your weight? How do you get off the diet hamster wheel? The answer -You will have to officially "break up" with dieting and DON'T GO BACK! Strive to move towards living a healthier lifestyle that will enable you to get better in all areas: physically, emotionally, and mentally.

Here are 5 steps to help you end your relationship with dieting[14]:

1. *It's not you, it's your diet.*

If you lost weight with a diet only to gain it back or you constantly reach a plateau (you can't lose any further weight for a very long period of time), you didn't fail at your diet–your diet failed you! About 95% of dieters gain all of the weight they lost and then some within 3+ years, and less for some.

2. *Don't forget the bad times.*

It's important to remember the bad times (when dieting) and all the reasons why you broke up with your diet. Anytime you think about going back to another "lost weight fast" gimmick, remember the time you weighed yourself after sticking to your diet and the numbers on the scale went up, and you were devastated for days. Remember all the guilt you felt any time you had something that was slightly off your diet, and the stress you felt about eating it afterwards. When you remember to focus on how difficult your

---

14 Poretsky, Golda, H.H.C. May 7 2012. "How to Break up with Dieting in 5 Easy Steps". http://www.bodylovewellness.com/2012/05/07/how-to-breakup-with-dieting-in-5-easy-steps/

relationship with your diet was, it'll be easier to not run back to the same gimmicks.

3. *Don't beat yourself up if you temporarily fail.*

We are human and it happens, so don't stress or beat yourself up for being just that – HUMAN. Change is not easy; as a matter of fact it can be downright hard, but it's necessary in order to grow and move forward. You may feel disappointed because you ate something completely unhealthy and the guilt consumes you. The lesson to learn is that it's okay if you temporarily fail, but don't stay there; get back up!

4. *Explore other options to meet your goals.*

Ever heard of the saying "there are more fish in the sea?" This is true even when it comes to changing lifestyle habits. There is more than one way to get to your destination. I purposely use the term "lifestyle" instead of just changing "eating" habits because this is exactly what it will take in order to sustain permanent change. This means changing the places you choose to eat (McDonalds® vs. Sweet Tomatoes/Soup Plantation®), people you socialize with (will they encourage you to stick with your goals, or enable you to revert to old habits?), the way you grocery shop (chip/cookie aisle or produce aisle?), and much more.

Exploring alternative options will help you figure out what foods, behaviors, environments, and exercises are really best for your body and your needs. For instance, if I know that I will be tempted if I drive by a Cold Stones Creamery®, then I know it's in my best interest to stay away from it!

5. *Your new lifestyle will become second nature.*

Over time, you won't miss living the old way because your body and mind becomes acclimated to the new habits. This means it's ok to take baby steps towards a complete overhaul. However, it doesn't mean you can never have another donut, a bowl of ice cream, or a piece of fried chicken again, but it does mean that you have learned to exercise control and moderation and can feel guilt-free to enjoy "fun foods" from time to time.

In a nutshell, diets are stressful, unhealthy, discouraging, and just downright a waste of time. By breaking up with all diet gimmicks, you will eliminate all the stress and guilt you experience around food and your body. Creating a permanent lifestyle change will cause you to think from a completely different place - where you will focus more on nourishment and what your body needs, and not so much on rules and restrictions.

DEPRESSION

It was a regular weeknight. I got home from work, threw my constricting work clothes on my bedroom floor and changed into a t-shirt and loose fitting pajama pants. I went into the kitchen and started prepping food for dinner that night (I'm sure it was something that was smothered, greasy, or fried), and in the interim decided to "treat" myself after a long difficult day at work to a pre-dinner bowl (or maybe it was a container?) of ice-cream.

I ventured into my family room and plopped down on the couch to veg out by watching mindless television. Scoop, click. Scoop, then click – I scooped heaping tablespoonful's of ice cream into my mouth as I clicked away with the remote control. "You can lose 10 lbs. in 2 weeks by drinking this shake!" Click… "By ordering today, you get 5 extra slim meals absolutely free!" Click… "And if you call right now, you'll get an extra 'burn that fat' DVD all for the price of $19.99!" Click… One weight loss gimmick after another.

Bored with everything I was seeing on TV, I decided to grab my phone to see what was going on in Facebook® world, only to scroll through my timeline with post after post of both men and women taking pictures of themselves in the gym mirror as they proudly boasted hashtags "#healthyliving" "#gettinitin" "#gettingmysexyback", and so on. "Good for them, but do they have to broadcast that they are at the gym every doggon day?" "Why do they have to post a pic of them sweating?" "Who cares if you're living a healthy lifestyle and working out!" is what I would say in my head over and over again as I scooped more ice cream into my mouth.

As I went for another scoop (the bowl was almost empty and I was thinking about getting another one), a small bit of the ice cream fell onto my right thigh, staining my pajamas. "Crap!" is what I thought; not because it stained my pajamas, but because I really wanted to eat that scoop! As I proceeded to wipe the ice cream clean from the light blue and grey fabric, I looked down at my thigh, I noticed that the width of it was almost as wide as the couch seat I was sitting on. "That can't be possible! Am I seeing this clearly?"… And more thoughts flooded my brain. I put the partially empty bowl down on the coffee table, and proceeded to look at how wide the stripes on my pajamas had stretched across my enormous thigh. It hit me like a ton of bricks. I had lost myself. I lied to myself. I pretended I was ok with the extra 40 lbs on my tiny frame. Now this might not sound like a ton of weight for some, but for an already 'curvy' woman whose only 4'11", 40 lbs. looked more like 400 lbs.

In 2003, I had lost around 20 lbs. through changing eating habits and exercise, then as fate would have it and with God's amazing sense of humor, I got pregnant in early 2004 with my second son Jalen. After giving birth to my son, I never did anything to lose the surplus weight again. I had not only regained the weight I lost from the year before, but added an additional 20 *more* pounds – just from eating and being lethargic! I realized it was at that point that I totally gave up hope. I weighed myself maybe once a year, and every year I watched the scale go higher and higher. "My weight's not too bad. I'm a mother after all. I just had a baby and I don't have time to lose weight. It's just 'baby fat'." Too bad my 'baby' was at the time almost 8 years old by the time I started noticing! I just kept eating and eating and eating. I enjoyed living a sedentary lifestyle – or so I convinced myself.

I hated the way I looked in the mirror, both naked and clothed. I did my best to avoid my reflection, and shopping for anything from the waist down was a nightmare! I felt like I looked like The Penguin character "Oswald Cobblepot" played by Danny DeVito from the movie *Batman Returns* - Short, extremely round, disgusting, and sloppy.

It didn't help that ironically, the Daytona Beach trip happened a week after my "thigh" discovery, adding insult to injury with me seeing my horrible reflection in the pizza shop window. I found myself slipping further and further into a deep depression; an emotional funk that I simply couldn't shake off. No one knew how I was feeling - not even my husband. I cried more within that 2 week span then I had in all the years combined. Even after the 2 weeks, for years I also found myself yelling at the most miniscule things (socks on the floor, a cup left in the sink, anything that the average person would overlook was magnified x 100 in my brain). I was constantly irritated (so much that I would even wake up irritated!), I was always pessimistic, my road rage was getting way out of control, and there were many times I felt like I was literally losing my mind.

I personally discovered that weight gain (or loss for some people) is highly linked with depression. What I was experiencing wasn't abnormal and I certainly wasn't alone. Why are depression and weight issues so connected? According to Dr. Joseph Hullett, MD, senior medical director for Optum Health Behavioral Solutions, "The part of the brain responsible for emotion — the limbic system — also controls appetite. When this emotional part of the brain gets disturbed in someone who is depressed, appetite gets disturbed as well."[15]

It makes total sense. Having weight issues (or even the perception of a weight issue) can be downright depressing. Being overweight fed into my self-deprecating 'I hate myself' thinking, which easily linked to depression. I also discovered after receiving thorough lab tests done that I also suffered from a severe Vitamin D deficiency – also linked to

---

[15] Hullett, Joseph, MD. August 3rd 2012. Major Depression Resource Center. "Weight loss Management for People with Depression". http://www.everydayhealth.com/hs/major-depression/weight-management-for-depression/

depression and weight fluctuations. It's a vicious cycle - you gain weight that contributes to the depression and also stems *from* the depression, then you may turn to food to self-medicate (numb the pain away). It's hard to get off the hamster wheel, but just because it's hard doesn't mean it can't be done!

Some of the symptoms of Depression included:

- Persistent sad, anxious, "empty" mood
- Persistent loneliness
- Restlessness irritability, excessive crying
- Feelings of guilt, worthlessness, helplessness, hopelessness, pessimism (this one was a doozy for me – I always saw the glass half empty).
- Sleeping too little, early-morning waking
- Overeating and weight gain
- Decreased energy
- Thoughts of death or suicide (thankfully, I don't have these thoughts any longer by the grace of God).

These were just some of the symptoms I experienced on a regular basis without even realizing that I was battling a heavier issue than just my weight. I recognized that in order for me to battle the weight demon, I had to first battle all of the internal issues that haunted me and would keep me from reaching my goals. It is an ongoing process that never ends –

constantly having to renew your mind isn't a one day event. I also understood that operating in wisdom and getting the proper medical help I needed to treat the chemical imbalance in my brain was also a part of the necessary steps I needed to take to be fully healed.

If you are battling with similar symptoms and need to seek professional help or medicinal assistance, DO NOT BE ASHAMED OR AFRAID to get the help you need to be made whole! There is no shame in exercising wisdom and getting the help you need to move you along the road to mental and physical health freedom. Since depression and weight are so closely linked, tackling both problems simultaneously is important to be able to move forward.

The following are some tips I used to help me conquer my fight with depression and weight gain:

1. ***Determine the relationship between the depression symptoms and eating.***

   I had to ask myself, "Why am I eating what I'm eating?" I had to figure out if I was eating because I needed to nourish my body, or was it because I was sad, angry, disappointed, bored, etc. I had to explore my feelings in relation to my weight and had to be mindful of how and when I used food as a crutch for deeper issues. Once I recognized the patterns, I was able to change them.

2. ***Don't Rush the Process.***

There were many, *many* days I felt completely overwhelmed with life in general, so instead of giving myself grandiose goals where I would beat myself up if I didn't accomplish them, I decided that having small, step-by-step weight-management goals was more important. Remember, there's nothing wrong with a baby step, as long as you step! I literally took it one day at a time, one step at a time. It can be as small as eliminating all carbonated drinks (all forms of soda) for a week. Once I accomplished that goal, I added another element to it the next week until I was able to kick the bad eating habits. This process also helped me not feel overwhelmed and was easy to follow.

3. ***Become more active.***

I have learned firsthand that not only does being physically active help you feel better about yourself and help towards weight loss goals, but it can also help ease symptoms of depression. In a study comparing exercise to antidepressants, they were equally effective at 12 weeks, and exercise was *more* effective at

10 months[16]. Amazing, isn't it? Bonus benefit – in most cases, exercise can be done for free! According to research from Mayo Clinic[17], regular exercise has many psychological and emotional benefits, such as:

- **_Build confidence._** Meeting exercise goals can boost your self-confidence. Knowing that you are progressively working on your health in itself can make you feel better about your appearance.

- **_Gives you a mental vacation._** *Exercise is a distraction that can decrease or even get rid of negative thoughts.*

- **_Become more social._** *Exercise may give you the chance to meet or socialize with others with a common goal. I have made new friends from around the world that I never would have made before through joining exercise groups.*

---

[16] Amen, Daniel G. MD. April 2nd 2013. "The Sane Way to Beat Anxiety and Depression". http://www.doctoroz.com/article/sane-way-beat-anxiety-and-depression?page=1

[17] Mayo Clinic Staff. 2016. "Depression: Major Depressive Disorder". http://www.mayoclinic.org/diseases-conditions/depression/in-depth/depression-and-exercise/art-20046495

- ***Ability to cope with stress.*** *Since exercise reduces stress, it helps with the ability to deal with life hurdles in a healthy manner.*

4. Obtain a thorough medical check-up.

This is a crucial step in your road to better health. You need to know the honest truth about EVERYTHING going on in your body – the good, the bad and the downright ugly. I discovered that my battle with depression and anxiety as a whole (I also had panic attacks for 9 years) wasn't just stemmed from being "overweight", but there were several chemical imbalances in my body that weren't being addressed.

Since I had hormonal problems I was totally unaware of that affected my mental health, it subsequently affected my physical health. It is crucial to get a full blown check-up from your primary care physician, to determine everything that's going on in your body to know the best solution to target the issue. Exercise in the natural is essential, but initially exercising wisdom is the key. Know where you stand first, before you start moving!

5. Prayer & Meditation.

Yes this sounds extremely cliché-ish, but I am a firm believer and a living witness in the power of prayer and meditation. I have learned that being a Christian doesn't exempt me from life challenges, but the exact opposite – I'm faced with constant challenges in my faith walk on a daily basis as a test of how strongly I believe in God. Although I have faced some of the most heart wrenching situations, I have never experienced a time when my prayers were not answered and my issues were not fixed. NEVER. Whatever your faith is, tapping into your spirituality can definitely benefit you naturally.

Why is that? It's a simple answer – for example: before I pray, I first check to see (in the Word of God) if what I am praying for lines up with exactly what God promised me as his daughter, and because I know with certainty that what I am about to pray is in total agreement with Him, I can then put a stamp on it that it will happen in due season. I can rest in knowing that it will be done, finished, completed, in *his* timing. It may not be when I want it to happen, but it is always when I need it.

You *can* permanently overcome depression, no matter how bleak your situation may seem. Remember this: don't beat yourself up for getting the help you need to move you to a healthier, happier life. Focus on what you can do, not on what you think you can't. You can do *faaaarrrrrr* more than you could ever imagine!

POINTS TO PONDER...

Dysmorphia or even dysmorphic tendencies is a real mental illness. It is also incredibly miserable to live day in and day out feeling as if you're inadequate. Constantly hating on your own appearance isn't healthy and causes more damage as time moves forward. If you need to seek professional guidance, please don't be ashamed or embarrassed to ask for the help.

Diets can be flat out discouraging. Even the mention of the word "diet" can immediately damper your mood. Creating a permanent lifestyle change will cause you to think from a completely different place – one where you will focus more on nourishment and what your body needs, and not so much on rules and restrictions.

Depression is a mental illness that MILLIONS of people deal with every day from all walks of life, yet countless will not seek the medical help they need out of fear, rejection, or embarrassment of being labeled as "crazy" (especially in the African American and Hispanic communities). If you are battling with similar symptoms and need to seek professional help or medicinal assistance, *DO NOT BE ASHAMED OR AFRAID* to get the help you need to be made whole!

CHAPTER 1
RECOMMENDED
"READS"

Dysmorphia

- ***The Broken Mirror: Understanding and Treating Body Dysmorphia Disorder,*** by Katharine A. Phillips, MD

- ***Understanding Body Dysmorphic Disorder***, by Katharine A. Phillips, MD

- ***The BDD Workbook: Overcome Body Dysmorphia Disorder & End Body Image Obsessions***, by James Claiborn & Cherlene Pedrick, RN

- ***Body Image Lies Women Believe: and the Truth of Christ That Sets them Free,*** by Shelley Hitz

Diet

- ***How Not to Die: Discover the Foods Scientifically Proven to Prevent and Reverse Disease***, by Michael Greger, MD

- ***Love to Eat, Hate to Eat: Overcoming the Bondage of Destructive Eating Habits,*** by Elyse M. Fitzpatrick

- ***What the Bible Says about Healthy Living,*** by Rex Russell, MD

- ***How to Have your Cake and your Skinny Jeans too: Stop Binge eating, Overeating, and Dieting for Good, Get the Naturally Thin Body You Crave from the Inside Out,*** by Josie Spinardi

Depression

- ***Bigger than Impossible: Keys to Experiencing the Impossible through God,*** by Lydia Chorpening

- ***Overcome Depression,*** by Matthew Mitchell

- ***Depression: 9 Simple Depression Self-help Steps to Overcome Depression for Life,*** by Otto Viteri

NOTES

Chapter 2: Numbers

"A good decision is based on knowledge, and not on numbers" - Plato

Our lives are dictated by numbers, all day, and every day. Go to bed at 10. Get up at 6. Step on the scale at 6:15 and see 255 lbs. Take a 5 minute shower while you cry over the 255 number for 8 minutes. Put on a size 16 dress, and a size 10 shoes. Cook breakfast for 2 kids at 7. Leave the house by 7:30. Pump $10 worth of gas because you can't afford $20. Go to lunch at 12 and eat 2 sandwiches, 3 cookies and 1 bag of chips. Drank 0 ounces of water, but drank 32 ounces of coffee. Worked for 8 hours. Back in traffic at 5. Picked up the kids at 5:30. Stopped by 3 stores and got home by 6:30. Took off the size 16 dress and the size 10 shoes. You decide to depress yourself even more by stepping on the scale at 6:45 and saw 262. Cried again for 10 minutes…

Numbers, numbers, numbers! Whether you like them or not, numbers play an important role in daily life.

Without numbers, you would have a hard time figuring out what time to leave for work or school, which interstates to take, or what size shoe you need to purchase. Without numbers telling you what the temperature will be, you'd be unsure on how to properly dress for the day. Numbers also allow you to determine how much you can spend on the things that you want (a new purse) versus the things you need (groceries). Numbers are neutral – they can be a positive and a negative, but at the end of the day, we *need* numbers!

Many people claim to hate anything involving numbers, especially math and statistics (and I was definitely one of those people!), however as much as we want to avoid numbers like the plague, we are ultimately dependent and obsessed with them regardless. We obsess with the numbers on the scale, numbers in our clothes, the number of calories we eat, the number of ranking we fall under at work, school or in a competition. There are even people who suffer with Obsessive Compulsive Disorder (OCD) who are obsessed with counting numbers!

Everyone carries a slight number obsession without even being aware. For example, using numbers to create a list transforms jumbled, unclear information into easy to process steps. When we see a numbered list, we know that the information we're about to read or hear will be easier to follow, understand, and should make more sense.

It's easy to conclude that "numbers" – which is a non-tangible noun, an arithmetical value, takes up a massive part of our world. Imagine going a single day without the use of numbers. It's impossible. Although we need numbers to survive, all of these unhealthy obsessions with numbers can be crippling and we are prone to become entrapped inside a numerical prison. In relation to weight, this is especially true for numbers on a scale, clothing, and calories.

SCALES

In spite of all the diet fads, fitness centers, workout videos, protein drinks, and workout equipment at our disposal, Americans (more than any other country) seem to still have the toughest time with weight loss and obesity. One of the main reasons for this struggle (and there are many), is due to an obsession with the scale.

A scale is merely "an instrument or machine for weighing".[18] Please get a clear understanding that the scale measures MASS, which includes

---

[18] Scale (n). Merriam-Webster.com 2016. http://www.merriam-webster.com/dictionary/scale

everything your body is composed: bones, fat, water, muscles, organs, and blood.

If you take nothing else away from this section, please absorb this - ***The numbers you see on the scale is not a precise measurement of your weight*** – just like your bank account balance from one day to the next doesn't measure your wealth. It consistently changes from one day to the next, from one week to the next, from one month to the other. One minute your up, and the next your down, like a roller coaster. The same applies when it comes to your weight and the usage of a scale.

Scales are designed to give you the mass weight of your body at the current day and time, and I have learned from experience that it should only be used as a referencing tool to stay on top of my overall weight and health, and not to define me as a person from one day to the next. My weight (and most people's weight – especially women) tend to fluctuate between 4-5 (or more) pounds throughout the course of the week. One day I'm down 2 pounds, but 2-3 days later I could be up 4 pounds. It varies based on my daily consumption, elimination, hormonal balance, etc. I have learned to only use it as a referencing point to make sure I am staying in a healthy range for my body. If by chance I saw the pattern changing (such as it's going up and up, week after week), then that's an indication that my nutrition and/or activity is off and I need to re-evaluate my behaviors and adjust accordingly.

Unfortunately, this is *not* how we are taught to use the scale. The multi-billion dollar diet industry thrives on primarily emphasizing on the number on the scale to define a person's weight loss progress. This can cause fear, obsession, and enslavement to the scale for many people who are uneducated in knowing how the body and weight really works. I was one of those people, and my goal is to help educate and debunk most of the myths to help you successfully become a healthier you.

For years, I started defining myself by what I weighed – so much to the point that I eliminated weighing myself for an extensive period of time and I cringed at the thought of being weighed. Knowing I had a doctor's appointment meant I had to be prepared to face the demon on the scale – that horrific number that was going to tell me exactly what I was worth and how much work I needed to do to get rid of it. Facing it meant I had to face my worst nightmare – my own failure reflecting back at me in a numerical format.

I have since learned that defining yourself explicitly by what you weigh can be the beginning of bigger emotional and psychological problems. It's like sliding into a vortex with no bottom in sight. It's a mind prison and can lead to a lifetime of yo-yo dieting, countless gym memberships, debt accumulation, and much more. But let's be real – you DO need to face the giant eventually. Not as a definition, but as a reference point so you know where you are and where you never want to be again.

In order to create a plan, you have to start with an agenda.

How do you know where you're going and how far you've come in your journey if you don't even know where you've started? It doesn't feel good. It's downright uncomfortable, and it's ok to shed tears (I have definitely been there and done that!), but once you get past the initial shock and disappointment, you can then take that small "scale" of information, and use it as one of the tools to help you accomplish your health goals!

 Let me paint you a picture of a bad relationship with the scale:

You find the latest "lose weight fast" trend and decide yet again for the 40th time that year to go for it! You're excited and revved about your healthy eating plan for days, or maybe weeks and demonstrate real discipline. You feel good about yourself, you're starting to see some physical changes, and you're giving it your all during your workout sessions. You get up one morning and notice that you're looking slimmer, and you immediately think to yourself – "Wow I'm doing great and I'm so proud of myself! I bet I've lost at least 5-10lbs!"

Then, without being properly educated, you decide to get on your bathroom scale to verify your thoughts. You step on with the hope of confirming that you've been killing it with your new diet fad and exercise, but then something terrible happens - the scale laughs back at you and almost taunts you as it proudly boasts that you haven't lost a single ounce or you've, in fact, *gained* weight? You're probably thinking, "What kind of voodoo witch craft is going on with this thing!" You step on and off, then on and off over and over while the number licks its tongue out at you, while you become more upset by the minute.

Your mood instantly catapults from elation to devastation, and you start second guessing all the choices you've made over the past few weeks. Where did you go wrong? What could you have done better? ....and your day is basically ruined. Even worse, you might have defeated thoughts such as, "What's the use? What's the point? Why am I wasting my time if it's not working?", then proceed to the nearest fast food place and get the largest, greasiest, most unhealthy thing on the menu you can find. A bout of guilt then flushes over you a minute after you've consumed it, and the tears begin to fall, the shame starts to creep in, and the vicious cycle starts all over again.

Does any of this sound familiar? Not only has this scenario happened to me countless times (more times than I can recall), but I have also seen it happen to family and friends as well. This is simply not the way the scale should be used! It is not the Alpha and the Omega, and it doesn't define who you are! It defines where you are in total body capacity at the time being, and should be used as such! Make a vow after reading this section that going forward, you will NOT allow yourself to continue to be a slave to a scale number, but to educate yourself with how your body works, and then use it as a tool to help with your weight loss goals, but not as your 'Messiah'.

So, what affects the weight you see on a scale? Here are the top factors that cause your number to change from morning to night, from day to day, and from week to week, etc.:

1. **Food & Drink**
   Every ounce of food and liquid you consume has weight. Think about it for a minute – when you look at the food packages, it even tells you how much the food or drink actually weighs (ounces, lbs., gallons, etc.). It even breaks down for you how much weight is per serving

(example: ½ cup of cereal to ¼ cup milk = 1 serving).

If your food and drink weighs something before you consume it, why would you not consider its weight once it's in your body? Even something as small as drinking a bottle of water can make a difference in scale weight because it adds to your overall mass. You weigh more when you have more waste. The more you eliminate, the lighter you typically become.

2. **Salt**
If you eat a diet high in salt your body is more likely to retain sodium, which causes unwanted bloat and water weight. Staying away from as much salt as possible will not only benefit your waistline, but your blood pressure will thank you as well.

3. **Hormones**
Especially for women - premenstrual hormones, stress, menopause, medications, all play a factor in the amount of water retention the body holds onto, causing extra body weight.

4. **Exercise**
Wait, what? Yes, even exercising can temporarily INCREASE your weight! All exercise, including weight training & cardio,

can cause muscle inflammation and water retention during the repair process. If you do happen to gain weight when you first start a new workout program, it's very common that your numbers will slightly increase due to temporary water weight caused by inflammation. Be patient, give it time and it will pass.

Understand that when you work out, it causes little tears in your muscle fibers that draws in the fluids in your body to repair itself that obviously weighs something. When inflammation is allowed to occur in a healthy way, it's temporary[19] and necessary in order to tear down and build up your muscles that eventually gives you a leaner, tighter appearance. Can you say sexy legs, arms and abs? Embrace the process knowing that whatever change you see on the scale from exercising is b/c your body is adjusting – AS LONG AS YOU'RE FOLLOWING THE PROPER EATING HABITS! Don't use this new found knowledge as a scapegoat if you're not eating properly.

---

[19] Faye, Denis M.S. July 21 2014. "4 Reasons working out can cause Weight Gain." Beach Body. http://www.beachbody.com/beachbodyblog/fitness/ask-the-expert-why-do-you-gain-weight-when-you-start-working-out

The above is only a few reasons the scale isn't supposed to be your #1 reliable source to determine your weight loss success, but you get the picture. So the golden question for the day is, **"If scales aren't so reliable, then why do we even use them?"** The answer is simply it's used as *A* tool, not as *THE* tool! No 2 scales are going to be calibrated the exact same way.

Use the scale as ONE method to track goals, but not as the end all answer. It's wise to use various means of tracking progress along with the scale such as measuring tapes, before and after pictures, and how your clothes fit.

TYPES OF SCALES[20]

There are so many scales on the market it's easy to become confused as to which one is the best one to use. While there are many styles and brands to select from, there are some key differences between scales that may help you determine which one will best fit

---

[20] Fitday. 2016. "The Four Best Types of Scales to Purchase". http://www.fitday.com/fitness-articles/fitness/weight-loss/the-four-best-types-of-scales-to-purchase.html

your needs. Below are the most common scales to date and how they work:

Balance Scale

Balance scales are the large, upright ones that you typically find in gyms and doctor's offices. You stand on a platform that uses a sliding balance mechanism. You move the weights around on the top piece until the scale is balanced in the center. Unless you have a good amount of space, can lift heavy weight (they weigh around 300lbs) and can afford it (approx. $200+), then this might not be the ideal scale to use at home.

Spring Scale (aka bathroom scale)

This is the standard floor scale that's been around for ages. It's small in size, allowing you to place it in your bathroom, bedroom, or anywhere you have a small space. How it works: You step onto it and your weight on the platform pushes down on a spring which then causes the disc to move. Gravity helps determine how far the disc needs to turn and a spindle points to your weight. They are known to be pretty reliable and fairly inexpensive. There generally is a dial, knob, button or other way to recalibrate spring scales on the side or bottom.

Digital Scale

With everything becoming digital, it's no surprise that the scale has also evolved. You can find these scales in the same size as the spring scale, making them convenient to have at home, but they can vary in pricing from a little (around $20) up to hundreds depending on the make, model and brand. You step onto the scale and your weight is calculated and shown on a screen. These are often battery powered and can read incorrectly when the battery is low. Since you are stepping on the scale, it measures similarly to that of a spring scale, only showing the result in a digital format. They have a reset switch if there is a problem with the scale.

BMI/Feature-Rich Scales

Since technology is so far advances, digital scales are now available with additional features that can give you more detailed information about your weight loss, such as Body Mass Index (known as your "BMI" or percentage of body fat), muscle mass, water content and more. These additional features offer a readout of results that greatly effects your overall weight. As you can imagine, this type of scale can vary in pricing around the same ranges as a regular digital scale. The more features involved, the higher the investment.

Remember, your weight can vary depending on the time of day, body water levels, and for women, hormones, menstruation and even stress levels.

Regardless of the scale you choose, the key is to make sure it works for your particular needs and is calibrated properly. If ever you find your scale doesn't seem to be functioning properly (despite calibration and comparing it to your weight on a scale at doctor or gym), consider investing in a new one to make sure that you're getting more accurate readings to help you with your weight loss goals.

CLOTHES

We've all been there before… you see the perfect outfit online, in the mall, or at your favorite department store, draped so cleverly over a size 2 mannequin and tightened in the back with a paperclip so it can accentuate the less than curvy figure of the Barbie doll mannequins' body. Your eyes sparkle; you can't stop checking out the design, the overall look, the feel of the material, and everything about that outfit screams "Buy Me"! You rush over to the rack to see if they have your size, and excited to see that they do! You grab it before anyone else can, and proceed to the nearest dressing room. You picture how absolutely gorgeous you'll look in it, and can't wait to see how it'll cling to your curves.

As you proceed to try and zip, button, pull up, pull down, and squeeze into the outfit, your excitement instantly turns into frustration, disappointment, embarrassment, and in many of my own cases, depression. The image staring back at you looked absolutely nothing like the image you pictured, and definitely looked nothing like that size 2 mannequin! Tears start to weld up behind your eyelids, and the positive thoughts you had when you walked into the store was immediately replaced with thoughts of defeat - "I'm fat!", "I look horrible in this outfit!", "That's it I'm going on a diet starting today!", "I can't believe how disgusting I look".... All things we have all said to ourselves at one point or another.

Newsflash! The clothing designers typically don't design around the average woman's figure, nor are the sizes from one designer to another exactly the same. There's a reason for this mental torture, and it has a history rooted in the evolution of industry standards vs. vanity over the decades. Why do you think within the most recent years that all mannequin displays are based as a size 0, 2 and possibly a 4? Vanity.

The increase of "vanity sizing" has deemed most labels meaningless, particularly in America. Over the years as Americans have started to balloon in size, industry brands have shifted their clothing metrics to make consumers feel 'skinnier'. Pretty deceptive trick, but it works.

For example, a women's size 12 in 1958 is now a size 6[21]. It has also become a bit discriminating, with most American women wearing a size 14, it's becoming increasingly harder to find, unless you directly shop from "plus size" stores. Think finding your true size is hard to find in stores? Then forget about trying to buy something online! I can't count how many times I've ordered something online and had to return it because the item was made for a small child instead of a full grown woman!

Yes I admit, I had a lot of work to do on my body for the betterment of my health and self-esteem, but there had to be some real explanation for why there were so many inconsistencies with all the clothing I tried on and failed to fit. Out of frustration and curiosity, I decided to do a little digging for myself to find out the scientific formula behind different designers thought processes on the sizing of their clothing. For a very long time until recent years, I knew right off the bat that certain stores were definitely a "no-no" for me based on the demographic

---

[21] Dockterman, Eliana. 2016. "Inside the fight to take back the fitting room". http://time.com/how-to-fix-vanity-sizing/

of their target audience, but even the stores I normally shopped were making it more difficult to find something that would actually fit.

For example, several years ago I bought a pair of jeans from one store that fit me like a glove. They were perfect in every way as if they were made just for me. I wore those jeans quite often because they gave me confidence, were comfortable, and were a nice design. Needless to say I wore them out pretty quickly, and proceeded back to the exact same store about a year later to buy a replacement pair.

I was super excited to see they still carried them, and proceeded to buy the same size as before. I got them home and tried them on (thinking they had to be the same as the others since they are the same pants), and I got a very rude awakening! The new pants were a whole 2 INCHES SMALLER than the original pair, but had the _exact same size labeling on the inside_?! I was floored. I held the new pants against the old pants and could instantly tell the difference. In order for me to get the pants I wanted, I had to buy a LARGER size, which I simply refused to do! The psychological torment such a simple thing as a number can cause is amazing.

The same way I felt terrible about having to get a larger size to accommodate the new industry standards, the polar opposite psychology is used to make women buy *more* clothes through vanity sizing. These companies purposely can turn a size 16 into a size 12 through the simple change of a size label, thus jarring women to feel good about themselves and buy more clothes. I come from a background with a lot of years in the sales and marketing industry, and this is by far one of the most creative yet deceptive and undetectable marketing ploys used. Retail giants bet on playing on a woman's emotions and know how sensitive most women are about their size and weight. Seeing the smaller number on the tag somehow gives validation. Sad, but very true. I have been guilty of falling prey to the marketing tricks the industry pulls to lure more money out of my purse. I'm sure I'm probably not alone.

I discovered that my experience with the jeans wasn't an anomaly. Take a look at the picture of the Gap® pants[22]. In 1996, the exact same khakis were a size 2, with a waist circumference of 28.5. Fast forward 10 years, the again the exact same pants were

---

[22] Triffin, Molly. November 12, 2010. "Vanity Sizing: The Insanity of size 0". http://www.cosmopolitan.com/style-beauty/fashion/advice/a3031/vanity-sizing/

labeled a size 2, but the waist was a whole 3 inches larger! The psychology of vanity sizing in full effect.

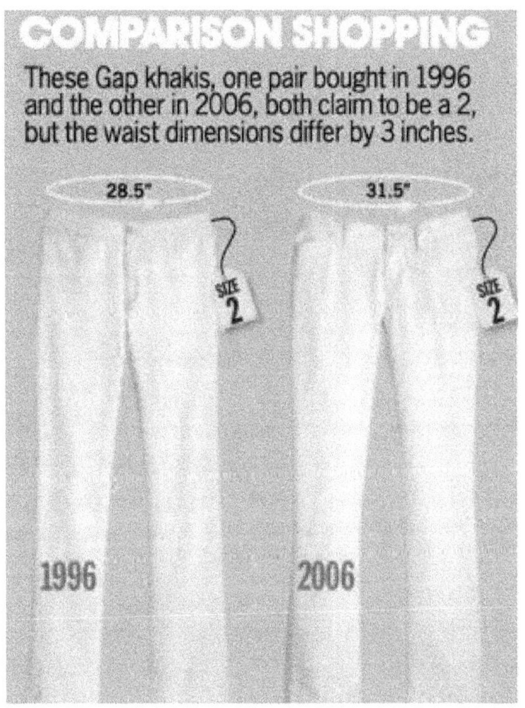

So the next time you see the perfect outfit that you just can't live without, remember the logic behind the numbers sown into the fabric. The numbers are based on a metric made by a vast array of designers that cater to a certain demographic. It's particularly harder to find a designer that caters to an African American or Hispanic woman's body. The numbers

DO NOT define you! While working on becoming a better you, understand that it's ok to temporarily buy what you need to make you feel beautiful.

I confess, I caved and bought the larger sized jeans after I realized the number in the waist didn't matter because it wasn't accurate, didn't define me, and didn't control my happiness. Don't let it control yours either!

CALORIES

Yep, more numbers! When does it ever end? If you're reading this book, I can probably assume that calories is something at one point or another you've glanced at on the side of the Cheeze-It® box to see exactly how many you can consume without feeling guilty.

While counting calories can be a helpful tool to in extent, it can also lead to dangerous behaviors if taken too far. To maintain a healthy weight and assist our bodies to properly function to survive, we need to consume a certain number of calories daily. The volume of calories needed changes whether you are trying to lose weight, maintain, or gain weight. For women the typical minimum of 1,800-2,000 calories per day is required to maintain a healthy weight, depending on physical activity level, age, and size.

For men, it's between 2,200-3,000 calories per day[23]. Calorie figures vary depending on the resource, so just take it as a generic example. Unless you are actively seeking to lose weight in a healthy manner, cutting below the bare minimum can put your mental and physical health at serious risk.

What is a Calorie?

Most of us have learned the science behind it in a grade school science class, but if you're like me you've used the term so much to where you don't even remember what it really is or how it affects our body. Calories are a *measurement of the amount of energy needed to complete daily functions*"[24] like breathing, resting and playing. Calories are also measured in food as a way to determine the energy content of that specific food.

Having knowledge of how calories really work and the benefits of different foods can help you avoid overeating as well as help maintain, lose, or even gain weight for some who battle with being under weight. While counting calories can be a very use

---

[23] Zelman, Katherine M., MPH, RD, LD. WebMD 2005. Diet & Weight Management. "Estimated Calorie Requirements". http://www.webmd.com/diet/features/estimated-calorie-requirement

[24] Szalay, Jessie. 13 November 2015. Live Science. "What Are Calories?" http://www.livescience.com/52802-what-is-a-calorie.html

tool, just like mentioned on the topic of scales, it is just a measurement tool, but not *the* tool! I have learned that it is so incredibly easy to tip the pendulum so far in one direction that you easily forget in order for it to function properly, it has to sway in both directions to have proper balance. Calories is just one point that the pendulum touches, but it doesn't stop there. Using calories in a healthy way is one of several tools that will help you become a better 'you'.

Like the numbers on the scale and the numbers in my clothes, the numbers in food had built yet another mental prison in my mind. Every single day, almost all day, I would think about how many calories every item I was about to eat had before I would eat it, and at times it would be virtually impossible to fully enjoy my food and my life.

It's a miserable place to be when you can't even go out on a date with your husband for the sake of worrying about how many calories is in the salad dressing, or to take your kids out and enjoy an occasional ice cream cone without feeling guilty and ashamed. I just flat out REFUSE to continue to be a prisoner to numbers of any kind, but to live my life to the fullest, and learn to enjoy the "not so healthy" foods within moderation. Hopefully you will also learn to adopt this mantra into your life as well. Like my oldest son once told me, "Mom ….LIVE!"

Here are 6 reasons to stop obsessing over calorie counting[25]:

1. **Nutrients Vary.**

Depending on the season, variety, etc. of the food, the calorie count will be completely different for a summer fruit that is sweet and ripe versus one that's out of season. There is no way for the USDA to analyze every single variety of every single fruit, vegetable, piece of beef, etc.

2. **Calories are *not* everything.**

Yes, calories exist, and if you eat too many you'll gain weight and if you eat too little you'll make yourself sick, but they aren't the entire picture. I could package up 100 calorie sticks of pure lard and tell you it's healthy because it only has 100 calories. Get the point?

3. **Labels are not 100% accurate.**

---

[25] Nichols, Lily RDN, CDE, CLT. 2014. "6 Reasons to Stop Counting Calories". http://pilatesnutritionist.com/6-reasons-to-stop-counting-calories-11-things-to-do-instead/

See the trend yet? Just like with designer industry companies who make our clothes, even in food packaging, there is a certain percentage of marginal errors on the nutritional facts panel allowed based on labeling laws. According to the FDA, *"The ratio between the amount obtained by laboratory analysis and the amount declared on the product label in the Nutrition Facts panel must be 120% or less, i.e., the label is considered to be out of compliance if the nutrient content of a composite of the product is greater than 20% above the value declared on the label."* (FDA Guidance for Industry: Nutrition Labeling Manual).

In other words, if a package says an item is "only 100 calories", it may truthfully be 119 calories, and this can be done <u>legally</u>. Shocking isn't it? It's yet another reason why you shouldn't get so caught up in numbers – they can be inaccurate at any given time.

4. **All calories are *not* created equal.**

Your body doesn't treat all calories the same way. High-quality calories come from nutrient rich foods like chicken breast, eggs, broccoli, leafy greens, grass fed beef, and healthy fats such as nuts and avocados – all considered LIVING FOODS. They make you feel fuller for longer periods of time and trigger fat burning hormones. On the flip side of the equation, foods that are very high in fat and/or processed sugar (fried foods, donuts, candy, processed meats, etc.) tend to trigger hunger at a faster rate, prompting overeating and absorption of more fat.

I know all too well how this works. I was a "sugarholic". I'm a baker by trade and I love what I do, but I've learned moderation is the key. Cakes, cookies, pies, ice cream, candy, you name it; I ate it and loved every minute of it! The more I ate, the more I wanted it.

Ultimately, my sugar addiction along with eating greasy processed foods led to me piling on over 40 pounds of unwanted weight. When I traded the exact same amount of calories I consumed when eating processed foods for foods that were nutrient rich, the weight started dropping. Switching to 1,500 calories of living foods versus 1,500 calories of sweets and processed foods made a gigantic difference in my overall health and waistline. Same amount of calories, but far from equal.

5. **Eating 1200 calories or less will make you skinny.**

False. On the contrary when you eat too little calories, you are starving your body of important nutrients and drastically slow down your metabolism. Guess what happens? You eventually start to store fat and burn muscle because your body goes into starvation mode. It doesn't know when it'll get the next real meal so it tends to hold onto the weight you have versus shedding weight. Your body is a machine and will act as such to sustain itself.

In my case, I started eating so little (close to only 750 calories per day!), and found that not only was I becoming weaker and more irritable, but I actually started to gain weight! Talk about being devastated and beyond frustrated. Everything I ate was being absorbed because I was robbing my body of the nutrients it needed to function properly. This is why those fad, restrictive diets mentioned earlier don't work. You may see some quick results initially, but because you never learned how to combine regular exercise and proper nutrition, the minute you start to eat like normal again, you tend to gain the weight you lost right back with extra pounds to follow.

Think about it this way – anything you get really fast without going through the process of learning, is bound to eventually fail. Ever heard of the cursed lottery winners? People who obtain a mass amount of money in one instant that didn't have 2 nickels to rub together the day before tend to struggle with going from one extreme to the next. Many of them end up right back to square one or in even worst state. Why? None of the financial lessons were learned along the way to know how to deal with acquiring that much wealth at one time.

The same lessons apply to your body. You simply can't believe that drinking shakes in lieu of meals, or in this case counting calories is a permanent, responsible way to become and stay healthy. How did I break my own cycle? By doing what you're currently doing – educating myself. If you know better you tend to be able to do better and feel better about yourself in the process.

6. "Low Calorie" doesn't mean "Healthy".

Don't let the clever packaging and brilliant marketing fool you! Many times opting for something just because it says "low calorie" or even "low fat" tend to have other hidden ingredients that are high in sugar or artificial ingredients, aka man-made crap. Instead of eating something a little higher In calories that's nutrient rich, you opt for the lesser calorie version that's full of junk that causes more harm than good. The ingredients list below came from a lite 50 calorie per serving salad dressing:

Water, balsamic vinegar, **soybean oil** and extra virgin olive oil, **sugar**, salt. Contains 2% or less of each of the following:

Spices, garlic powder, **caramel color, xanthan gum, sodium benzoate** and **sorbic acid and calcium disodium edta** (used to protect quality), **propylene glycol alginate,** gum arabic, **natural flavor,** sulfur dioxide.

The items in **BOLD** represent not so healthy elements - laboratory preservatives that are easily overlooked because if it's "low calorie", it has to be the better option.

The Bottom Line - When you make a real lifestyle change by eating healthy foods and incorporating regular exercise, you don't have to be consumed with counting calories. As long as you give your body what it needs, it'll take care of the rest. So learn to relax! This is something I had to tell myself and continue to tell myself on a regular basis. Focus on quality over quantity. High quality foods include non-starchy vegetables (leafy greens such as spinach & kale, zucchini, green beans, mushrooms, etc.), nutrient-dense proteins (eggs, chicken breast, fish, beans), and whole-food fats (avocado and almonds). Guess what they all have in common? No labels!

Not sure how to break free from the calorie counting cycle? Consider doing some of the following:

- **Listen to your body.** If your body is saying it's starving, but your brain tells you that you can't be because you just ate a measly 300 calories at lunch, LISTEN TO YOUR BODY!

- **Actually take time to sit down and enjoy your food.** Stop eating on the go or in a rush and allow your body to naturally become satisfied. Eating in a rush typically lead to picking unhealthy options and poor digestion, leaving you feeling hungry a lot quicker than if you sat down to have a real meal. If you have to eat while multitasking (which I often have to do because of my business), take some time and prep healthy on the go meals and snacks.

- **Make a conscious effort to choose healthier foods that don't require any thinking.** No, salad is not the only thing you have to eat for the rest of your life! There are literally hundreds of healthy, delicious recipes for you to try that actually taste great. Some of my favorites are actually included at the end of this book!

- **Be realistic.** There is nothing wrong with having an _occasional_ slice (or 2!) of pizza, a hot piece of crispy fried chicken, or a warm, fudgy brownie sundae. The key is **moderation**. Life would absolutely suck if it wasn't for the small pleasures to enjoy. Learn to make this type of eating the exception, and not the norm... Learn to LIVE, and live guilt-free!

POINTS TO PONDER…

You Are Not Defined by a Number. EVER.

Don't get caught up in numbers so much that you can't focus on what's truly important – your health and how to feel about yourself. Again (and this is being repeated on purpose so you get a real grasp of understanding) - your weight fluctuates so much from day to day, and the scale should only be used as a guide, not the be all and end all. Ask yourself – at the end of the day, which is more important: how you look, feel and perform, or what a lifeless, brainless scale tells you whenever you step on it?

Remember what's Important.

We all want to be healthy, feel confident, and perform our best in life, both inside and outside. Obsessing about the weight on a scale can actually hinder and even halt your weight loss goals. If after reading this you still find yourself stuck on the number on a scale day in and day out, it may be time to set some new goals that don't revolve around the scale, such as using a tape measure to track your inches lost, working on dropping a pants/dress size, or buy something really nice in a smaller nice, and when you can put it on, you'll know that you've made progress! Start using the scale again once you've shown yourself that is doesn't define your success.

At the end of the day, the scale number doesn't measure your worth as a person, which could never be measured.

It's ok to strive to be better and do better, but extremes can be unhealthy, miserable, and ultimately lead to overall dissatisfaction and unhappiness. Don't do what I so often did – reach a goal and still didn't feel satisfied. I would harshly critique myself and belittled the small progress I was making, all because I wasn't receiving the validation I felt I needed from a number.

Something I have to remind myself daily: Psalm 139:14 (NLT) ***"Thank you for making me so wonderfully complex! Your workmanship is marvelous--how well I know it."***[26] So no matter where you are on your healthy journey, you are wonderfully made and irreplaceable. Even more important - Your worth has no numerical value!

---

[26] Psalm 139:14. The Holy Bible. New Living Translation. BibleHub.com http://biblehub.com/psalms/139-14.htm

CHAPTER 2
TOP RECOMMENDED "READS"

Scales

- ***It's Not About the Scale: Weight Loss Motivation: 7 Steps You can Take to Never Diet Again…and Love Yourself Skinny,*** by M. Rathstone

- ***Tipping the Scale: How to Make Peace with food and your when Dieting no longer works***, by Lara Zuehlke

Clothing Industry Standards (Websites)

- ***"The Psychology of Vanity Sizing"*** by Roger Dooley. 29 July 2013.Forbes.com http://www.forbes.com/sites/rogerdooley/2013/07/29/vanity-sizing/#116e08f76831

- ***"Vanity Sizing: The Insanity of Size 0"***, by Molly Triffin. 12 November 2009. Cosmopolitan.com http://www.cosmopolitan.com/style-beauty/fashion/advice/a3031/vanity-sizing/

Calories

- ***"The poor, misunderstood calorie: calories proper (Volume 1)"*** by Dr. William Lagakos, Ph.D.

- ***Good Calories, Bad Calories: Fats, Carbs, and the Controversial Science of Diet and Health,*** by Gary Taubes

NOTES

Chapter 3:
The "F" Word

"Food is the Most Abused Anxiety Drug; Exercise is the Most Underutilized Anti-Depressant." –
Unknown

Let's be real. Life can make it incredibly hard to take care of ourselves the way we should. Life gets in the way— work, kids, spouses, significant others, parents, other relatives, school, businesses, and the list goes on and on. When faced with the choice between doing what's right versus what's convenient, 9 times out of 10 we choose what's convenient, myself included.

Regardless of whether it's convenient or not, maintaining our health should automatically come first. We have only ONE body, and if we aren't healthy, we can't fulfill everything in life we are purposed to complete. Sadly we take our health for granted; many of us until it's too late.

I am guilty to the fullest extent. There were many days when I would be stuffing my face with the latest fried concoction or the newest supersized meal and knew I was wrong. I was slowly cutting off days from my life – all for a quick food "fix". My flesh was screaming for more, while my brain and heart was screaming "Stop!" It was a vicious cycle. Every time I thought about getting my life together and becoming healthy, there were 3 'F' words in the back of my mind (and no it's not the infamous profane one) that kept me stuck in a rut: **Food, Fitness**, and **Frustration**.

FOOD

Boy do I love food! Mexican, Italian, seafood, good ole southern comfort foods, you name it, I love it! To top it off I'm in love with sweets – cakes, pies, cookies, donuts, ice cream…ummmm hmmmm! D-E-L-I-C-I-O-U-S! Food is just one of those things in life that gives us so much pleasure, but can also lead to a lifetime of pain if not properly handled.

In my family everything revolved around food – birthdays, 'just because it's Sunday', 'we woke up', 'I stumped my baby toe', 'bought a new car', any reason at all was a good enough reason to fry something up! Not only did my family tend to lean on food a great deal, but all foods were improperly prepared: carbs on top carbs (is it really necessary to have rice AND a loaf of Wonder bread® on your plate?), fried everything (pork chop, chicken, steak, fish; heck – I think we even fried ice cream once or twice!), gravy smothered, doused in sugar or salt (collard greens in my house was more like sugar w/collard greens!), or slathered in grease. Even vegetables in my house were cooked so long that there was no nutrients left in them. Needless to say I didn't learn the best eating habits as a child, and as a result my parents had to buy my private school uniforms in the "husky" section. Even as a kid I knew it didn't sound right.

Have you ever had a transparent conversation with yourself about your relationship with food? I say "transparent" because not only do we lie to others, but we lie to ourselves. I was a habitual liar to myself. I knew I had a serious problem, on top of dealing with low self-esteem and being very self-conscious about my appearance. Yet, I kept telling myself every time I wanted to eat something terribly unhealthy that "there was nothing wrong with me", "my weight wasn't that far out of control", "just one more donut won't make a difference", "I might as well be fat and happy", and the biggest lie of all – "I just can't lose any weight", and the list of lies go on and on. Denial to the 10th degree.

Once I really started getting raw and honest with myself about how I truly felt, I was able to gather the courage and strength I needed to make some drastic changes. I had enough. I was tired of not loving what I saw in the mirror. Tired of dreading the torture of shopping for any clothes, and sick and tired of constantly feeling unattractive, unhealthy, and defeated. The first step in my decision to make a drastic change was to get a revelation of my relationship with food and my associated behaviors when it came to eating.

I discovered that the primary reason I ate was because of boredom and because it made me feel better about whatever situation I faced. I also noticed I never ate breakfast, resulting in constant snacking of the wrong foods through the day. Although I typically didn't overeat, the things I chose to eat were very unhealthy when I did. Top that with living a very sedentary lifestyle (almost zero exercise) alongside a terrible metabolism, and it became the formula for a perfect storm of weight disaster.

I know I'm not the only one that's had a love/hate relationship with food, and more times than I can count I've been in the hate relationship corner (feelings of guilt, shame, frustration, anger, etc.). If any of this sounds like you, I'd recommend you take the time for at least 1 week to:

1. Write down how many times you eat per day.
2. What food choices did you make?

>3. Why did you make them? (Were you scared, bored, lonely, or actually hungry?)

This is how I discovered that I ate a great deal out of sheer boredom, and rarely did I eat because I was actually hungry. I also found myself eating late at night and grazing randomly throughout the day. Once you get a hold of the "Why" you do what you do (a.k.a. the ROOT of the issue), then it's much easier to execute a plan to help you overcome poor eating habits.

Here are some suggested questions to help you get started:

1. Am I eating because I am hungry or am I eating because it is "time" to eat, i.e. breakfast? Lunch? Snack? Dinner time?

There were times I ate simply because it was "time" to eat although I wasn't hungry. I just ate out of habit. Yes, we should follow a set schedule to keep our bodies regulated, but to eat to just "eat" is a different story.

2. Is this food really going to nourish and support my overall wellbeing or is it being used to soothe something deeper?

A large slice of chocolate cake topped with 2 scoops of vanilla ice cream tastes great, but it adds very little nutritional value to my body. Again, there is nothing wrong with an occasional treat, but this was a choice I made all the time – something sweet, greasy, or salty to make me "feel good" about whatever was going on at the time.

3. What is my intention behind eating this?

My intentions was to solve whatever issue I was having at the time – stressed, boredom, need for attention, need for affection, numbing depressive or suicidal thoughts, and the list continued.

4. What Feeling Am I Trying to Get From Food?

Food was my antidepressant and my friend. It never turned me down, never disappointed me, and never made me feel less than good enough. All it ever did was make me feel great – for the moment.

5. Is This Physical Hunger or Emotional Hunger?

When I asked myself this question, I found that about 80% of the time I was eating out of sheer emotion. Dealing with all the internal issues I carried made me turn to food as a crutch to sooth my emotions.

6. Is This Physical Hunger or Emotional Hunger?

Believe it or not, although I was eating, I discovered there were times when I didn't eat all day long and then binged later in the day on everything I could grab. I also found that because I wasn't eating the right foods my body was malnourished. That's one of the biggest myths, that if you're obese or morbidly obese then you're not malnourished. In most cases it's the exact opposite because the body isn't getting the right nutrients it needs to properly function.

Junk in, junk out - this includes what you drink. I was one of those people that despised water. I hated the very thought of drinking it over other sugary, fruity, delicious drink options. My primary beverage of choice was fruit juices and an occasional soda. Once I started changing my lifestyle, I discovered that I was severely dehydrated.

7. Is This Physical Hunger or Emotional Hunger?

Almost every time I ate I immediately felt guilty and ashamed of myself. It felt great going in, but the minute it was gone, the negative emotions started to come in like a flood. It's such a bad feeling! Just like any other drug, to get rid of the bad feeling I had to eat something else to make myself feel better. It was a vicious cycle.

8. Is This Physical Hunger or Emotional Hunger?

Folks, let's make something crystal clear – What you allow yourself to see, hear, feel, etc. over an extended period of time and exposure, WILL seep into your real life whether fiction or nonfiction. We are humans built with senses.   Ever saw a commercial or social media post about an amazingly delicious slice of pizza and found yourself thinking about ordering one? We don't buy food with our feet but with our eyes first! It's how we are conditioned. Be very mindful of what you allow to sit in front of your eyes.

I can't count how many times I went and bought something scrumptious I saw advertised or got up off my couch and walked into my kitchen to make something all because *the idea* was planted in my head through what I encountered. Make a note of how many times you've seen food advertised and how many times you've thought about eating it. Then think about how many times you went through with your thought?   Take the time to cut back on the amount of time you spend (especially on social media) watching recipes, restaurant menus, etc. to decrease your chance for sabotage and temptation.

First thing's first: **Free yourself.** Your body cannot give you what you need when there is constant emotional despair. Since the human body is a machine, it takes on all the negative banter and manifests it into STRESS. Stress can turn into heart disease, blood pressure issues, ulcers, and other diseases. Your body cannot function optimally when there is such stress and turmoil.

Start freeing yourself from marrying negative thoughts and feelings with your food by doing the following:

- **Stop punishing yourself for what you ate yesterday (or even today!).** You ate it, it's gone, now move forward! Learn from your mistakes and keep it moving. You are not perfect.

- **Slow Down and Eat: sit, chew, and enjoy your food.** When I took the time to slow down and actually digest a meal, I found that I was satisfied quicker, didn't overindulge, and my brain was able to signal my stomach that I was full.

- **Let go of the need to be perfect.** You're not and never will be, so stop beating yourself up over a slip-up every now and then. After all, like my son reminded me - you do have to live! I am a tried and true "perfectionist". I am extremely hard on myself when I don't do something 150% right and it's been a battle for me to accept that it's ok to not get it right all the time. I have learned to give myself some leeway. Give yourself a "free day" that you can enjoy whatever foods you like _in moderation_. I typically give myself a "free meal" instead of an entire day because my body doesn't do well with a full day of bad eating habits any longer. You have to do what works best for you and your body.

- **Stop comparing!** What works for Chantelle, Jason, Christine, Eric, Tasha, and Kimberly may not work for you! There is only one 'you' and your body is uniquely yours! Yes, for the most part our human bodies universally function the same, but everyone has different needs according to their own physical make-up.

Stop assuming that because Tasha was able to lose 10 lbs. in 1 week (which is beyond unrealistic) by eating grass and air while drinking vinegar that it will work for you too. Stay in your lane and do what works best for your body! Don't get me wrong - It's very hard to not compare. It's an ongoing practice to keep reminding yourself that what works for you may not be what works for the next person and vice versa. It takes time to figure out how your body functions so you can make educated decisions on the best regime for you.

- **Remember: You only have ONE body!** No explanation needed.

Tackling your relationship with food is the largest part of the battle. The secret to real, lasting weight loss is knowing the formula: 80% diet / 20% exercise[27]. You simply cannot exercise away your weight problem with terrible eating habits. It just doesn't work. The 80/20 ratio is controversial to say the least in the health and fitness world… some say it's more or less in either direction, but I've found personally that it fit the bill for my particular needs.

So exactly how does it work? According to Dr. Albert Matheny, R.D., C.S.C.S. co-founder of SoHo Strength Lab and PROMIX Nutrition, *"The key to weight loss is achieving a negative energy balance, or taking in less calories than you burn,. To shed a single pound, you need to achieve a 3,500 calorie deficit. So if you're following the 80/20 ratio, you'd*

---

[27] Gomez, Alexandria. 1 August 2016. Women's Health. "Is Weight Loss really 80 Percent Diet and 20 percent Exercise?" http://www.womenshealthmag.com/weight-loss/weight-loss-80-percent-diet-20-percent-exercise

want to burn approximately 750 calories through exercise and cut an additional 3,000 calories through dieting. You don't need to hit an exact 80/20 ratio to shed pounds, but it is important for people to focus primarily on diet when they're trying to lose weight. "You can lose weight without exercise, but you cannot lose weight if your nutrition counteracts your energy expenditure through exercise," explains Dr. Matheny.

Below is a visual example of what it looks like:

LOSING WEIGHT WITH 80% DIET AND 20% EXERCISE		
DAY	**EXERCISE (CALORIES BURNED)**	**CALORIES CUT THROUGH DIET**
MONDAY	250	600
TUESDAY	0	600
WEDNESDAY	250	600

THURSDAY	0	600
FRIDAY	250	600
TOTAL BURNED	**750**	**3000**

The total amount of calories burned is 3,750 for the week which is typically a <u>1lb loss</u>. Losing 1-2 lbs. per week is a safe and doable goal with the right habits in place. Remember weight loss and lifestyle changes are a journey, *not* a sprint!

The reason dieting is so much more effective than exercise is because it takes a ton of activity to create a 500 to 700 calorie deficit through working out. Essentially, "you'd need to run 7 to 10 miles a day to lose one pound a week", says Holly Lofton, M.D., an assistant professor of medicine and director of the weight management program at New York University's Langone Medical Center. The average person can't keep this up, especially without increasing their caloric intake.

"I see this in patients all the time," says Lofton. "People think, 'If I run the marathon or start going to boot camp, I'm going to lose weight' but they're often disappointed when they don't." Simply put, it's virtually IMPOSSIBLE to think you can eat the exact same way (as many of the fad diets suggest), and lose weight by exercise alone. If your lifestyle doesn't change, neither will your waistline!

In spring 2013, when I finally decided to take my lifestyle change very seriously, one of the first things I asked myself, "What would be the most *extreme* workout to help me jumpstart my journey?" At that time, it was none other than at-home workout DVD *Insanity®* instructed by Shaun T, created by Beach Body® (www.beachbody.com). No, I don't work for Beach Body nor am I endorsing their products, however, I felt using at-home workouts would allow me to feel free to work as hard as humanly possible to get into shape without the thought of 900 humiliating eyes watching me in the gym. I needed something that would challenge me to no end, and that's exactly what I got with the *Insanity* workout!

Within the first 5 minutes of the fitness test, I almost passed out (not even the actual workout but the test)! I cried and cried because I couldn't believe how far gone I had allowed myself to get, and how horrible shape I was really in from being so sedentary all those years. Nevertheless, I refused to quit. I did as much as I could, when I could, and eventually I felt myself getting better by the day. Working out at home also gave me the freedom of getting it in when I had the opportunity, instead of making up excuses for not going to a gym. I had to use what worked best for me and my schedule, therefore please feel free to do the same for you, whether it's workout at home, working out at your local park, getting a personal trainer, joining a gym, or going to exercise classes. We all have to start somewhere. No one gets to the middle and the end of the road through thin air.

One of the major takeaways that I learned when I started the program was how to pick the right foods to fuel my body. Beachbody developed a food category breakdown called Michi's Ladder® (it's pretty similar to the USDA food pyramid that we're all familiar with seeing, but with much more detail) that makes it very easy to know what foods to eat heartily, which foods to each moderately, and which foods to stay completely away from altogether.

According to Beach Body, Michi's Ladder® consists of five food tiers, with tier 1 considered the highest tier and tier 5 considered the lowest. The Michi's Ladder is based on the Japanese term "michi," which means "the way." Basically, the ladder shows you "the way" to eating a proper diet without all the guess work. The foods in tier 5 include items high in calories and fat and low in nutrients. As you climb towards tier 1, you'll see low-calorie, low-fat foods that contain high amounts of vital nutrients[28].

---

[28] Michi's Ladder. 2017. https://www.beachbodyondemand.com/blog/nutrition

Followers should focus on foods from tiers 1 and 2, and avoid foods from the other tiers as much as possible. The more you choose to eat from the "clean" tiers (1&2), the healthier, leaner, and more energetic you should become. Following this tool made it much easier for me to pinpoint foods I can indulge from time to time (tiers 3-5), and foods I should be consuming on an everyday basis (tiers 1-2). This is merely a *tool*, something that I am introducing to you that has worked and still works for me. There are countless tools available that can fit your lifestyle, so do what works best for your dietary needs.

For illustrative purposes, the following table is a sample of foods that would fall under each tier, so you can get the idea of which foods to eat liberally, and which foods to eliminate. You can find an actual tier model by visiting the Beach Body website and typing in "Michi's Ladder".

TIER 1 (BEST)	TIER 2 (BETTER)	TIER 3 (GOOD)	TIER 4 (WAR-NING)	TIER 5 (STAY AWAY!)
Apples	Banana	Plain Popcorn	Bagels	French Fries
Avocado	Blueberries	Applesauce (sugar free)	Hot Dogs	Donuts
Beans	Zucchini		Potato Salad	

Broccoli	Tortilla (wheat)	Baked fries	Spaghetti w/meat sauce	Cakes/Cookies
Strawberries	Peaches	Chicken Taco	Fried Fish	Alcohol
Egg Whites	Plums	Shrimp	White Bread	Bacon
Salmon	Hummus	Potato (baked or broiled)	Popcorn w/salt &Butter	Nachos
Kale	Black Coffee	Sushi		Sugared Cereals
Sweet Potato	White meat chicken	Low Fat cream cheese	Pork Chop	Coffee Creamer
Collard Greens	Nonfat Cheese	Unsalted Butter	Pretzels	Onion Rings
Tomato	Farm raised fish	Almond Milk	Cobb Salad	Buffalo Wings
Romaine Lettuce	Turkey Breast	Refried Beans	Ham	Fast Food Breakfast Sandwich
Onions	Veggie Burger	Hard Cheese	Ground Beef (20% fat)	Beef Taco
Oatmeal	Nonfat yogurt	2% Milk	Graham Crackers	Gravy
Olive Oil	Water-melon	Lamb	Sloppy Joe	Cheese-burger
Citrus fruits	1% Milk	Ketchup	Tuna Salad	Ice Cream
				Pot Pie

I have learned and continue to learn that when trying to make a lifestyle change it's not going to happen overnight. Take baby steps; one day at a time to learn how to eat less C.R.A.P. (carbonated drinks, refined sugar, artificial foods, processed foods), and eat more F.O.O.D. (fruits & veggies, organic foods, omega 3 rich foods, drink more water!)

Remember, making even small changes can drastically reduce your waistline and increase your lifespan. Make a commitment to make at least ONE change by the end of this chapter and start it right away. Give yourself at least 21 days/3 weeks (the amount of days it normally takes to break a bad habit) and see how far you've come. Everyone is different so if it takes you longer, so what! Just keep moving forward.

FITNESS

Exercise. Work-Out. Fitness. Regardless of which term you use, unless you're a hard core athlete who enjoys rigorous activities, exercise (especially for beginners) is HARD! It can be dreadful, painful, stressful, uncomfortable, and will put your physical, mental and emotional capabilities to the biggest test.

It makes you sweat, stink, swell, and can make you downright delusional. These are the things that most fitness experts *won't* discuss, but it's reality for a person who goes from sitting on the couch scrolling their phones on social media to getting up and becoming physically active.

I was that person. I was the person who hated seeing people on Facebook® post about how they went to the gym and "blah blah blah". I was the person who despised seeing those dumb weight loss commercials. I was sick and tired of seeing those annoying Zumba® fanatics post video clips on Instagram® of how "awesome" their class was that day. Everywhere I looked, I was being crammed with images and words from people doing exactly what I KNEW I should be doing – getting my behind off the couch and getting my mind/body/soul together.

I just didn't want to admit it. I didn't want to admit I had an eating problem. I didn't want to admit that I was not okay being the size I was at that time, and I definitely didn't accept myself. I didn't want to admit that I was insecure, embarrassed, and ashamed of what I had allowed myself to become. I couldn't handle the thought of admitting that if I even tried exercising, that would mean putting on clothing that would show every fat roll, every imperfection, every stretchmark, and every cellulite dimple that I had been hiding under my clothes for years. I didn't want to admit that I didn't want to face the truth; because I couldn't handle the truth - I hated me. I hated how lazy and sluggish I had become. I hated admitting that I hated everything about myself. Facing the exercise giant would mean that I had to face the real Goliath in my life: ME. All I knew at that time was that I finally had more than enough of the pity party, and either I was going to get up and do something about it, or I was going to continue to sit on the couch, and be angry, irritated, and annoyed at everyone else for doing what I didn't have the strength nor the courage to tackle.

Once I made up my mind that enough was enough, I had to take the larger picture and break it down into small puzzle pieces, so I wouldn't feel so deeply overwhelmed with the large task at hand. I have learned that no matter what obstacle in life you face, if you handle it in smaller increments, it becomes easier to endure. Exercise is no different. Here are some very helpful tips that worked for me when I initially started on my journey (and still apply to this day):

1. ***Learn from Past & Present Mistakes***. There was one thing I knew for certain – what NOT to do! Rehashing what worked and what didn't work for you in the past is the easiest first step you can take towards finding the right regimen. I remembered all the lack of success I had with certain types of work out programs, and some I just couldn't stand to do for various reasons: way too long, too fast, too hard, or just plain boring.

   Whether you're just beginning, in the middle, or have reached your fitness goals and currently maintaining, it's inevitable that you *are* going to make mistakes. The trick is to pay attention to these mistakes and learn from them. The better you understand your shortcomings, the better you'll be able to find what works best for you. You'll be able to tailor your workout program to your own needs. This means better results in the future and the ability to actually stick with your goals long-term.

2. ***Make Exercise a HABIT.*** Going to the gym one time is definitely a great start, but you

won't see changes in your mind and body unless you make it a habit. Pick a time in the day to dedicate strictly to you! Even if it's only 15 minutes in the morning or 30 minutes after work, you _must_ make your exercise time sacred from all people and all circumstances! Fitness Experts say that the best time to work out is first thing in the morning, so you don't come up the with excuses as the day gets busy, as well as kick start your metabolism for the day.

I've done both morning and evening workouts, and I've found that yes, it is way easier to make an excuse in the evenings to not work out after a long day, but I also discovered that when I came home from work, it became a stress reliever and helped me unwind. Once my schedule changed and allowed me to switch to working out in the mornings, I discovered that I was more conscience about my food choices throughout the day (because I didn't want to 'undo' all of the work I put in that morning), as well as gave me a sense of accomplishment that it was already done for the day. Whatever works for you, work it into your routine!

Life will continue to happen, but it's up to you to take full charge over your health and wellness, which means "they" (whoever your "they" may be) can wait 15 minutes, 30 minutes, or however long you have to devote to yourself. Don't get stuck on trying to do an hour long routine that you already know you're going to quit after 10 minutes.

If you know that realistically all you have to give physically is 10 minutes, then find something that will make you give your ALL for that 10 minutes! Stop making things harder than they have to be and start thinking smarter. Naturally, as the days and weeks go by, you'll find that you're able to do more, have more energy, and what you initially started out doing isn't going to be as much of a challenge. That's when you push yourself to do an extra 5 minutes or add something harder to the routine. This is called making *progress*! However there's a catch - You'll only see progress if you <u>maintain consistency</u>! If you give up at the first sign of discomfort, you'll be right back to square One. Any progress is better than zero progress!

As a mother, it is incredibly difficult and can even feel guilty to take time away from the kids, your spouse, or anyone or anything else that requires our constant attention. Believe me, THEY WILL LIVE! The earth will not stop spinning because you decided to put yourself first for a change. In fact, by taking the time out to take care of yourself, you're actually prolonging your longevity, your sanity, and your quality of life which will positively affect those around you. As an example, initially shoot for working out 3 times each week for the next three weeks. Pick a schedule you know you'll keep such as Monday/Wednesday/Friday either morning or evening (whatever works for you), for the allotted time you want to devote. Building lifelong habits takes time, but once you've built those habits into your daily schedule you'll notice that when you miss doing your workouts it'll feel weird and abnormal.

3. ***Educate (and keep Educating) yourself!*** You will <u>never</u> reach a point of knowing it all! Once you believe you do know it all, you've already failed. It's important to not only read this book, but to read other books, articles, blogs, or anything else that will continue to renew your mind, assist you with setting new habits and goals, and to keep you motivated and encouraged.

4. **Get a Cheering/Motivating Section.** One thing I have learned in my lifetime is toxic people can pass on toxicity. Make a decision

today to remove any people from your circle that will hinder your progress in any form. You simply have no room for pessimistic, consistently negative, downright belligerent people in your life while you're trying to make changes to improve yourself.

Surround yourself with those who are genuinely happy for your decision, and even better – find someone or several people who are on a similar journey as yours, and band together to keep each other motivated and encouraged! Initially, I didn't have anyone cheering me on once I decided to live a healthier lifestyle. I was on my own, and found out very quickly that it's very lonely to pursue change and have no one to push me when I didn't feel like pushing myself. However I got creative with finding support – I went online and joined weight loss support groups, and had the opportunity to virtually meet people that helped me stay focused on my goal, and most of all, they could relate to my journey.

5. **Ask Questions/Ask for Help.** You simply can NOT do life alone. No one should isolate themselves and be on an island without any help. If you don't know what to do, have lost control and have slipped back into old habits, start feeling depressed, need advice on

exercises, or anything that might come up during your journey, don't be afraid to reach out for help and ASK! Lay all pride and embarrassment aside and seek the assistance you need! You can ask your healthcare provider, your mentor (I strongly suggest you get one if you don't have one!), your spiritual leaders, your motivational group, fitness instructors, or anyone else who you see fit to assist you with getting the answers you need to be able to keep moving.

6. **Lose the Monotony.** This was a tough one even for me to stop. I'm a perfectionist. I like things done a certain way and I like having a planned schedule with a planned routine.   I found myself making myself stick to a certain workout plan that I absolutely hated, all because I had embedded into my brain that if I started it, I needed to go ahead and finish it, no matter how boring or ineffective it was for me. I realized that all I was doing was making myself miserable and that I wasn't enjoying the process. Once I freed myself from the mental prison of having to be "perfect" all the time, I was able to switch off the monotony button.

I started seeking after those workouts that were fun and effective at the same time, that I actually looked forward to doing instead of whining and complaining. For example, I love to dance! I've always enjoyed dancing even as a little girl, so I decided it would be beneficial for me to find workout routines that incorporated dancing. I still did my regular hardcore workouts, but I also learned to relax and switch them up from time to time with dancing to make the task more enjoyable. Lately I've switched from dancing and have found a new love for boxing and speed walking outdoors.

My point is – you don't have to feel stuck in a rut of doing the same ole routines, or using the same equipment in the gym, etc. It's ok to switch it up to keep your interest. Even more important; keep in mind that your body is a machine. Once it's programmed to do something, it easily gets acclimated and the effect of what you once did, will no longer yield the same results. Your body will go into "plateau" phase (where your body is staying in the exact same place), is this is VERY frustrating stage in losing weight. For this reason alone it's a good idea to change up your routines to keep your body "surprised".

7. **Listen to your Body.** Your body will tell you when something isn't right. If you're working

out 7 days a week nonstop and giving your body no time to recuperate, or even the opposite – if you're not working out at all and your constantly sluggish and lethargic, your body is telling you it needs something to change! Give yourself some leeway to learn what works for your body and what doesn't and listen to it. If you have a workout that is way too strenuous and your knees feel like giving out, then stop doing it! Find something else that is less taxing on your knees and keep it moving. The point is to find what works for you, but exercise wisdom in everything that you do.

8. **Don't Believe the HYPE!** You **cannot** just exercise your way to a slimmer, sexier, healthier body ***if you don't change your eating habits***! If your idea of losing weight quick, fast and in a hurry means eating whatever you want and taking a placebo pill to make you think it's blocking all the fat and carbs in the food, you can forget it! In order to sustain a healthy lifestyle and get to (and STAY) your ideal weight goals, you MUST permanently change your eating habits. The best way to get healthy and stay healthy is to make a permanent lifestyle change that includes a balance of proper eating habits with a combination of regular exercise.

When it comes to fitness, there are so many options on the market that it can make it overwhelming to decide what would work best for you. Most people immediately think of joining a gym, or joining a workout class, while others would rather run or walk, and others prefer to work out at home through virtual routines. Whatever you find works best for your schedule, make a consistent effort to JUST DO IT. Start small and work your way up to new levels and learn to challenge yourself to do better each time. Remember, doing something (even if it's only 10 minutes to start), is way better than doing absolutely nothing.

FRUSTRATION

It's inevitable, you WILL have moments of total frustration. Change SUCKS! That is, change that requires complete cooperation, discipline and sacrifice. Change that's uncomfortable never feels good, but without it there is no progression. It's mandatory that you learn to embrace the process of change and keep your focus on the end results!

Here's the truth – our bodies are created to need 4 major items to function:

1. **Food** (meaning Living foods that help nourish, clean, and protect our body).

2. **Exercise** (and no, you don't have to work out like a fitness maniac 7 days a week at 5 hours a day!)

3. **Rest**. Surprise! Losing weight and/or becoming healthier is NOT going to happen if you are not getting the proper rest. Also, say this word with me "v-a-c-a-t-i-o-n". Vacation isn't a "luxury"; it is necessary to regroup, relax, and get rejuvenated!

4. **Water**. I don't care how much you try to substitute drinking water with sports drinks, juice, sodas, etc.; nothing will ever take the place of water. How important is it? You can generally live 3-6 weeks without food, but you can only live a maximum of 7 days (more typically 3-4 days) without water.[29]

Notice that nowhere on the above list is: Pills, wraps, shots, hormones, meal plans, diet shakes, etc. I am a firm believer that as humans we have the tendency

---

[29] Spector, Dina. 14 May 2014. "How many days can a person survive without water". Science Business Insider. http://www.businessinsider.com/how-many-days-can-you-survive-without-water-2014-5

to make things way more complicated then they need to be, and we have the innate ability to blow circumstances way out of proportion. Weight loss is no different. I'm definitely not exempt from being guilty of doing way too much to accomplish a goal that could have been completed much sooner had I just slowed down and simplified the process. It's our distorted perception that leads to the utter frustration. We sabotage ourselves without even knowing it.

But despite the obstacles you will face on your journey, whatever you do, DO NOT QUIT! Quitting just isn't an option. From the undesired food choices, to crowded gyms, to your *extremely* sore muscles, the feeling of frustration will eventually pass. I like to say you have to just 'press through the pain to get to the gain'! As with anything, pushing through in the beginning is always the toughest part. Oh, and did I mention that you'll also try to convince yourself that the old 'you' is just fine? I can recall at times when I felt like I was torturing myself that it wasn't that bad being overweight. I might as well just be "fat and happy" then "fit and miserable", blah blah blah. LIES!

As fast as I was myself lying to myself, I quickly remembered the feeling I had every time I looked in the mirror. I remembered crying in dressing rooms because none of my old sizes would fit. I remembered the insecurities, low self-esteem and feelings of defeat. When it gets really hard, when you don't want to eat another salad, and when you're simply tired of being tired, here are three reasons why you should keep going despite the temptation to quit:

1. **Don't see results? RELAX! The results will come**. We live in such an "I want it now!" microwave mentality world that we just can't stomach the thought of actually _waiting_ to see the results of hard work. Patience is key. It often takes time for your body to adjust before your transformation happens. Although it can be hard, with persistence you can break old habits and your resolution will become a lifestyle. Once you get into a routine and stay consistent, you will start to see results.

2. *You're doing something right if your body is sore.* If you aren't experiencing any soreness, you aren't pushing yourself out of your comfort zone. Being sore is your body's way of letting you know that you're working hard. Know that the aches are temporary and a sign of achievement! However, if the pain seems too intense or lasts longer than a couple of days, seek medical advice to make

sure you're not suffering from an injury. *It is also crucial that you seek the permission of your physician before starting any exercise program to ensure it is safe for you!*

3. **Overwhelmed or Need Accountability? Find a Workout Buddy!** Starting anything new can be very intimidating. If you're starting to feel overwhelmed by exercises, how to prepare food, proper workout clothing, or any parts of the process, ASK FOR HELP! I realized that I needed to find someone to go through the process with me, find a support group, or something that could help push me along the way.

I managed to "buddy" up with another friend that was on the same path, and discovered that I wasn't alone, and had made way more progress than I realized. My perspective had drastically changed. Going at anything alone makes for a long, miserable process. Finding a support system always makes any task much easier to tackle.

Here's some additional advice: DON'T OVER DO IT! In the beginning of my journey I found myself going way overboard. Working out 2 hours a day 7 days a week, not allowing my body to rest, not getting enough sleep, undereating (basically starving myself out of fear that I'd reverse my progress), was actually sabotaging my progress. It's just as important to take a mental break from working out just as much as a physical one. Without it, you risk burning out, which can get in the way of you reaching your goals. Believe me, I've been there.

Signs that you are doing way too much include:

- Exhaustion. Exercise should make you feel better, not worse. If your mood is low or you feel lethargic, you could be seriously overdoing it with the workouts. Scale it back a bit to regain your energy. Being exhausted will only hinder your workouts, not help them.

- Sleep Deprivation. If you work out too much, it could be interfering with your ability to fall and stay asleep.

- Constant soreness. Yes, when you are first starting a new exercise program will be sore for a couple days or even weeks which is normal, but if the soreness last longer than that, you could be over doing it.

I know exactly what you're thinking. You're afraid that taking a day off will turn into two or three days and then you'll lose your motivation and slip back into old habits. However, if you burnout from overexerting yourself, you're more prone to throwing in the towel. To avoid burn-out:

- **Take 1-2 days off each week, especially in the beginning.** Instead of doing your full workout routine, consider just doing stretches on your off days or simply rest! I typically worked out 2-3 days then took a day off, then another 2-3 days and another day off. Some people work out 5 days straight and take 2 days off, etc. Do have to do what works best for you, but rest is necessary for your body to rebuild.

- **Vary your workout intensity.** Doing hardcore workouts every single day is a sure fire way to burn yourself out. Different variations and degrees of intensity will not only help you avoid burnout, but help you avoid boredom! Also, after a while of doing the exact same thing your body will become acclimated. This was one of my biggest issues – acclimation. The minute I would get a routine down, I found that my progress started slowing down because it was no longer a challenge, which leads to the next point –

- **Vary your workout program.** Changing your routines will not only improve your ability to see results, it'll alleviate boredom, prevent burnout, and help you use your muscles in a variety of different ways so you can fight off acclimation. That means you have more fun and see better results. I have consistently changed my routines. One week I may do speed walking, while another I may do a mixture of hip hop dance and boxing. Do what you enjoy, but mix up the routine.

Yes, there will be days that you'll want to give up due to frustration. At those times, take a moment to settle your mind and remember the purpose of your transformation. Even pictures of a healthier version of yourself will help keep you motivated. Remember the reason for the journey in the first place. Remember your "WHY"!

POINTS TO PONDER…

Regardless of whichever "F" word you endure, understand that life will continue to happen, and the earth will continue to spin. In other words, there is never a "right time" to start eating the right food, there is never going to be a "perfect time" to start your fitness routine, and there will certainly never be a time when you won't have to face frustration.

Life gets in the way— but it's totally up to YOU whether or not you decide to allow obstacles, trials and tribulations to stop you from living your best life possible. How we choose to live our lives is a matter of cause and effect. The causes may not always be in your power to control, but you certainly can control the effect.

Whether you know it or not, you have total dominion over your thoughts and your actions. Make a commitment today to start implementing actions that will make the "next" you, better than your "now" you!

CHAPTER 3
TOP RECOMMENDED "READS"

Food

- *"Food Can Fix it: The Superfood Switch to Fight Fat, Defying Age, and Eat your Way Healthy",* by Dr. Mehmet Oz

- *"It Starts with Food: Discover the Whole30 and Change your Life in Unexpected Ways"*, by Dallas & Melissa Hartwig

Fitness

- *"Thinner, Leaner, Stronger: The Simple Science of Building the Ultimate Female Body"* by Michael Matthews

- *"Bigger, Leaner, Stronger: The Simple Science of Building the Ultimate Male Body"* by Michael Matthews

- *ACSM'S Complete Guide to Fitness & Health 2nd Edition* by Barbara Bushman & the American College of Sports Medicine

Frustration

- ***"The Frustrated Dreamer: When your Dreams are Bigger than your Now"*** by Juanita D. Jones
(For the Mental, Spiritual and Emotional)

- ***"Downsize: 12 Truths for Turning Pants-Splitting Frustration into Pants Fitting Success"*** by Ted Spiker & Dr. Mehmet C. Oz
(For the physical)

NOTES

Chapter 4:
Body Talk

Have you ever scrolled through social media, watched a T.V. show or movie, or even walked through a shopping center and instantly started comparing your physique to those you perceive as being "perfect"? If you honestly answered 'yes', then you're certainly in good company.

We have the tendency to gravitate to features that we feel are perfect for what we'd want for ourselves, and it's so common for us as "normal" people to compare ourselves to celebrities we see on big or small screen. I had to realize that I couldn't (and shouldn't) compare myself to someone who paid for their curves, their flat belly, and their flawless, cellulite-free thighs.

There is simply NO WAY a woman can be pregnant, give birth, then a week later posing for half nude photos completely wrinkle, stretch mark and fat-free! Hollywood will have you believing that there is something seriously wrong with YOU (especially women) if you don't look like a Sports Illustrated ® centerfold a week after having a baby. We are all unique, and we all have different body types that determine how weight loss or weight gain affects us genetically.

The average person doesn't have a clue what their body type is, and the science behind how to work within your body type to create a healthier 'you'. The goal of this chapter is to educate you in layman's terms regarding the different body types, so you can identify which category you fall within, in order to be equipped to work with a program that best designed for *your* body (and not some propaganda version of a fantasy, factory made version of a body).

We can thank (or not thank) our genetics for our body reactions from certain foods, our strength as well as our weaknesses, and behaviors that we're predisposed to that we either struggle with or gifted. Have you ever noticed that some people are just naturally skinny, naturally fat or naturally muscular? It's not your imagination. Believe me, I've come across those people that seem to eat everything in sight and won't gain a pound, but if I even *smell* a cheeseburger I'll gain 10 pounds!

Different body types play a role in how easy or hard it is to change how our bodies look. Once I learned where I stood in regards to my body type, I was then able to properly tackle it the right way. Some people *(ectomorphs)* seem to eat whatever they want and never gain weight – the people I despised! Some people *(endomorphs)* seem to gain weight no matter how much they workout or how little they eat. Last, some people *(mesomorphs)* look like they workout, even when they don't (a.k.a. "the perfect body").

After testing, I discovered that I was originally all Endomorph, but then after changing my lifestyle I landed in between 2 body types – Endomorph and Mesomorph. You can actually have traits of more than one body type! But what this meant for me is I had to work extra hard to lose weight, stay far away from refined sugars, and I needed to have a serious love affair with weight training in order to change my natural body tendencies of holding onto fat. Genetics is something we just have to live with whether we like it or not – it just is what it is. Fortunately though, we don't have to be stuck forever being in our natural body types. With hard work and the desire to change, we can transform our bodies into the healthiest state possible.

Below a quick breakdown of each body type. See if you can identify which category(s) you may fit:

ENDOMORPHS

Endomorphs are typically people with wider waists, large bone structures, and are predisposed (by those pesky genetics) to storing fat instead of building muscle. They also have the tendency to struggle to lose weight despite drastic dieting and rigorous exercise.[30] These are people who were likely always a little bit bigger than everyone else most of their lives. I certainly can relate to this body type. As a kid, I can recall always shopping in the "chubby" sections of the Zayre®, J.C. Penney® or Morton's® clothing stores.

As an adult, I discovered that despite trying every diet on the market or trying every new fad workout, I seemed to gain weight just thinking about food and found it nearly impossible to lose it and keep it off. However, just because this body type is more prone to weight gain doesn't mean it can't be changed with discipline and hard work. I'm a living witness. Unfortunately, it's the genetics of an endomorph that make it a whole lot harder to reach a weight loss goal, especially when compared to the other body types, but it <u>can</u> be done!

---

[30] "The 3 Body Types Explained: Ectomorph, Endomorph & Mesomorph".   Taken   04   December   2017. http://www.directlyfitness.com/store/3-body-types-explained-ectomorph-mesomorph-endomorph/

Common Endomorph Traits:

- Slow metabolism
- Naturally lacking tone or leanness.
- Thick bone structure
- Typically have large appetites (loves to eat)

The cold, hard truth: If you identify with these characteristics, you might need to be more careful with consuming refined sugars (cakes, cookies, candy, soda, etc.) and processed foods (chips, boxed dinners, etc.) than other people, as you might be more genetically prone to storing those foods as fat rather than burning them as fuel. However, ***you also can NOT utilize your body type as an excuse or a crutch for not doing something to change it.***

One thing I have discovered throughout my fitness journey is you can work out until you pass out, but as stated before, WHAT YOU EAT will be responsible for 80-90% of your success or failure when it comes to weight loss. Yes, it's not fair that you can't eat everything you desire at any given time, but to reach your health goals, you'll have to learn to swallow this hard pill in order to move forward with a plan of attack. Believe me, I'm speaking from experience! You just have to implement the "3 P's": *proactivity, persistence and perseverance* to get the results you desire.

ECTOMORPHS

People who are classified as Ectomorphs have the tendency to be small framed, long, thin, and have low fat storage. They aren't predisposed to neither build muscle nor store fat, which is why regardless of how much they eat, they can't seem to gain any weight.

I know several people who fit into this category, and believe it or not, they HATED with a passion being so small. The way I felt about being so thick is the exact same way they felt about being the opposite. These are men and women who were more than likely very thin their entire lives without having to put any effort into their diet or workout.

Common Ectomorph Traits:

- Extremely fast metabolism
- Small bone structure/skinny
- Have the tendency to be fidgety
- Often picky eaters
- Naturally lack muscle tone and strength

Ectomorphs battle with the exact opposite genetic factors that endomorphs have – it's extremely difficult for them to gain weight and build muscle, and although it is possible for them to develop a slightly thicker frame, due to genetics they will only get but so built.

MESOMORPHS

These are the folks that have the best of both worlds. They are neither fat storers like endomorphs, nor do they have a problem with putting on weight/muscle like ectomorphs. This is the body type we fantasize about - not too thick, not too thin; just enough muscle tone and perfectly proportioned. These people are truly blessed genetically. The people that fit into this category are typically fitness models, body builders, athletes, and are often naturally muscular and lean without putting any time or effort into a diet or workout.

Common Mesomorph Traits:

- Ideal metabolism (not too fast, not too slow)
- Naturally lean (regarding muscular physique versus "skinny")
- Naturally athletic
- Ideal bone structure (not too thin, not too thick)

If your desire is to have the "perfect body", your goal (without you even knowing it) is geared towards the characteristics of a Mesomorph. I was amazed when I tested to find out my body type that I was actually a combination of Endomorph (thick framed, easily stores fat) AND mesomorph (because although I am thicker, I am hourglass shaped and have the ability to be lean (through hard work of course).

However, it was only within the last few years that I was able to change my body type from being completely Endomorph to a cross body type to "Endo-Meso". You can also test yourself through several websites available online. Simple search for "body type test", and you'll be able to get a very good indication of where you may fall.

Don't let your body type be an excuse!

So why did I feel it was necessary to go over such boring science jargon regarding body types? You don't know what you don't know, but once you do, you have the ability to change it! This is exactly why everything advertised doesn't work universally for everyone. This is also why so many people become agitated and frustrated that nothing seems to be working for them. It's not a "one size fits all" when it comes to all the weight loss/gain gimmicks. Eye-opening, isn't it?

Believe me, when I found out my body type, I was better able to work with a plan that was designed for

MY BODY, not for the lady who's been fit her entire life. Ever notice how all of the workout videos tend to have all super FIT trainers teaching? How about the cast working out with them? ALL totally fit! It's not relatable to the person who's struggling to even do 1 pushup let alone 20 (that was me!). It's just rare in the health and fitness industry to see "real" men and woman represented, which is the entire point – to sell you a dream, and it works! The diet industry is a multi-BILLION dollar business, yet in the US, we are getting fatter and fatter. Breaking the cycle of ignorance by educating on how our bodies work, and offering insight on real solutions on how to truly become healthier is the ultimate goal I pray you find within the pages of this book.

Regardless of our body types, we can still get the results we want – with HARD WORK! I'm sorry to tell you that it doesn't come in the form of a bottle, or shake, or waist trainer alone. Aids are good to help with jumpstarting, but it comes down to old fashioned effort and a complete overhaul of eating habits. Yes, our genetics will make certain things harder for us (unless you're blessed to be a mesomorph). However, that doesn't mean they prevent us from becoming our best.

BODY IMAGE

Let's briefly revisit scales, numbers, and how weight works. I know I'm not alone when it comes to being a prisoner of the scale, believing that those 3 numbers that show up represent my full worth. It takes time to reprogram your thinking from believing that you should obsess over a machine that weighs E.V.E.R.Y.T.H.I.N.G in your body – not just "fat". As stated in chapter 2, most scales are not designed to tell you everything that's going on in your body, leaving you naturally assuming that the full number appearing is a glaring replica of how fat (or how skinny) you really are, resulting in either a feeling of defeat or triumph.

The problem is one minute you're excited, and the next minute you're a ball of emotions. It's never ending. But in reality, how much a person weighs doesn't actually reflect their level of fitness or health status. Our genetic make-up, body type, and for women- menstrual cycles or the hormonal effects of menopause, water retention, gas and bloating (even from eating healthy foods), digestive problems, are only a few of the items that contribute to the average person gaining about 3-5lbs throughout the day. You can't gain 5lbs of "fat" in one weekend, and you can't lose 5lbs of fat in one weekend – no matter what the "box or the bottle" claims!

Keep in mind when you hop on the scale and see it up one day and down the next, it isn't accurately monitoring your progress. Ask yourself how do you feel in your own skin? Are you losing INCHES (which is what truly matters)? Are you becoming leaner and building more muscle in place of fat? Again, I'm not a "scale rebel" that's going to tell you to throw away your scale forever. Remember, it's to be used as an indicator tool ONLY (meaning it's great to use as a gauge so you don't get out of control), but not to be used as the gospel truth of what's really going on in your body

Did you know that not everyone carries weight the exact same way? Different body types carry weight in totally different directions. Take for instance the following photo of six different women – all from different background, religions, and nationalities.

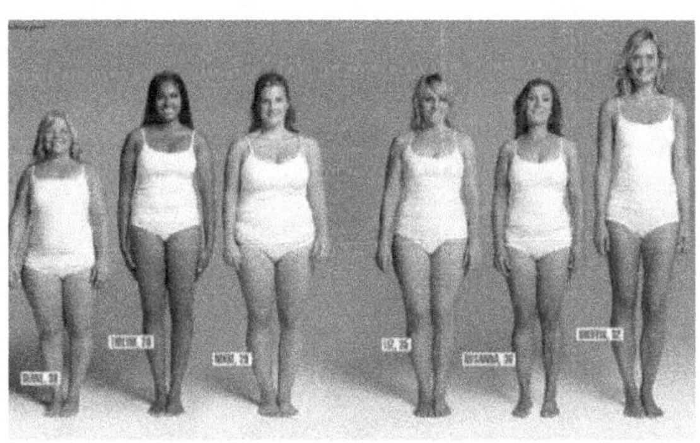

They are all different heights, different shapes, and they represent all 3 body types (endomorph, ectomorph, and mesomorph). What could they possibly have in common other than all being female? Believe it or not, they ALL WEIGH THE

SAME! Every woman pictured if exactly 154lbs[31]. The point? Learn to fit into your own mold. Take for instance the woman on the right (tallest) in comparison to the woman on the left (shortest). They both weight the exact same amount, but the tallest women wear a size 8/10 dress, while the shortest woman wears a size 12/14 dress. If the shortest woman tried to squeeze herself into the size 8 dress, she would instantly feel inferior and defeated – but they weight the EXACT SAME. This is why it's silly to compare your body to someone else's body. Your goal should be to become the absolute best YOU, not the best 'them'.

Here are some other examples of what different bodies look like with different make-ups:

---

[31] Johnson, John and Krista. 2017. "All these woman weight the same". Fit By Faith. http://www.fitbyfaith.net/motivational.html

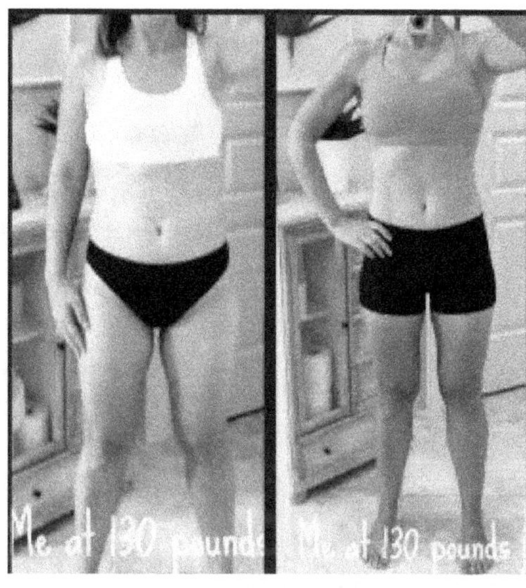
Me at 130 pounds
Me at 130 pounds

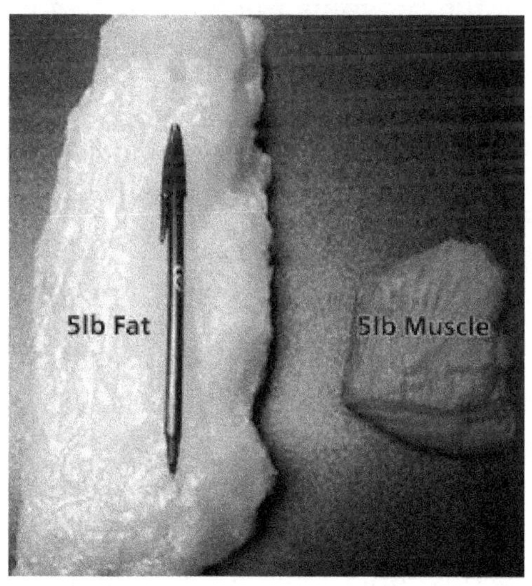
5lb Fat
5lb Muscle

As you can see, the woman in the picture shows that at the beginning of her health journey she weighed 130lbs. The woman in the picture on the right is the SAME WOMAN several months later after hard work and dietary changes, and weighs guess what: 130 lbs! Although she didn't lose a single pound from the scale, her total body composition drastically changed.

As you can see in the photo next to the woman, the fat on the left represents her 'before' picture, and the muscle on the right represents her 'after' picture. Let's make one thing clear: Contrary to what you might have heard or have even said before: **Muscle does <u>NOT</u> weight more than fat!** A pound, is a pound, is a pound! There are no different "pounds" of anything. However, muscle is DENSER than fat, which means it takes up much less space, thus giving a leaner, tighter appearance.

Is it making any sense why the scale does NOT represent the progress that's truly being made? The woman weighs not a single pound less, but lost countless inches, converted her fat reserves into muscle, and wears 3 sizes smaller than before.

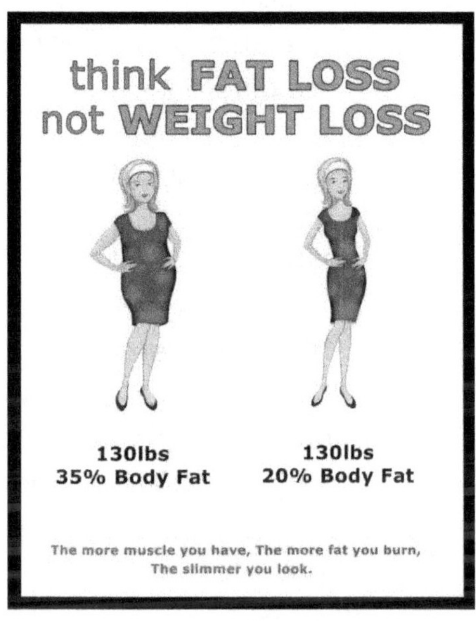

The above poster mimics exactly what happened with the woman in the other picture. Although she weighs the same, she looks and feels completely different. I can attest to this same scenario. In 1998, I weighed about 130lbs, but wore a size 10 in pants and dresses and was totally out of shape. I couldn't do 1 push up if you paid me. Fast forward after babies and life happening, I ballooned to about

180lbs in 2011, and wore a size 14 (and was heading into a 16). After making the decision to fully change my lifestyle, I dropped to 145-150 range (it fluctuates), but I wear a size 4/6 in dresses and size 7/8 in pants. Notice the difference?

1998: 130lbs size 10

2011: 180lbs size 14

2017: 145-150lbs size 4-8

Although I weigh more than I did in 1998, my body composition is completely different (more muscle definition), resulting in a leaner physique. Here's something else you should also understand: According to the US weight calculation chart used by most doctor's offices, at my height (I'm a petite woman at only 4'11"), I should only weigh between 95lbs (yes, you're reading this right!) to 125lbs MAX.

Based on their chart, I would be considered OBESE! How absolutely INSANE does that sound? By the way, the chart is EUROPEAN based on Eurocentric body frames, and does _not_ take into consideration that different ethnicities (African American, Hispanic,

Asian, etc.) tend to have completely different body frames based on genetics, thus the medical world has decided to measure every single person against a bias chart. How can a woman who's lean, completely healthy (zero health issues whatsoever), and wears between sizes 4-8, be considered "obese"?

I can easily state that at 95lbs, I would look like I was suffering from an eating disorder or a major drug problem. Even at 120lbs, I would still look sickly and unhealthy. I am simply not built to fit into American society's measure of the "ideal" weight.

Regardless of your muscle mass, or whether you're an athlete or an average citizen, the American system of weight measurement (whether it's with the chart or through the use of Body Mass Index or BMI) isn't as universal as it's been promoted to be over recent years. According to the chart, athletes who are thicker like Serena Williams would be considered 'Overweight' or even 'Obese', because her body weight would measure heavier because she is extremely lean. There's been a great deal of debate over the last few years regarding the use of the bias weight charts as well as BMI measuring because it doesn't take into account age, gender and race, which has led to falsely identifying certain ethnicities (especially African American) people as 'overweight'. This type of system of health assessment can be detrimental to anyone's psyche who may be battling with self-esteem issues (like I did), and can actually lead to unhealthy eating habits and even eating disorders – all for the sake of fitting into an unrealistic box that wasn't designed for all people in the first place.

So, the next time you go to the doctor and they whip out that totally biased chart, you will now be educated enough to know that more than likely if you aren't of European decent, it wasn't designed for you in the first place and carries zero 'weight' (pun intended) on how truly healthy you are or how you feel about yourself. Exercise wisdom and common sense. You certainly know when you're truly overweight/obese versus trying to fit into a perception of what's "healthy". I am comfortable in my own skin, all of my medical lab results across the board are superb, and I'm happy with my appearance. THAT is what matters!

POINTS TO PONDER...

Your body is uniquely YOURS. There is only 1 "you" and everything about you was created and designed for a purpose!

Regardless of how thin, thick, short, or tall you are, <u>everything about you is amazing</u>! Yes, you may have things that you want to change and need to correct, but nothing about how you was created is a mistake.

Disregard the nonsense that society tries to coerce you into believing on a day to day basis with pseudo-physiques that are unrealistic, plastic, and airbrushed.

STOP MAKING COMPARISONS to body types that are not like yours! Identify with *your* body type and work to become the absolute best YOU, not the best "someone else".

Ditch the dumb numbers! Focus on what really matters – fat loss instead of just focusing on what the scale says, and your overall health and wellness instead of what a bias weight chart states.

CHAPTER 4
TOP RECOMMENDED
"READS"

"Compared to Who?: A Proven Path to Improve Your Body Image" by Heather Creekmore

"Body Kindness: Transform Your Health from the Inside Out—and Never Say Diet Again" By Rebecca Scritchfield

"Dr. Berg's New Body Type Guide: Get Healthy Lose Weight & Feel Great" by Eric Berg Alexandria

NOTES

Chapter 5:
The Journey

This book isn't just 6 chapters by mistake. Each chapter represents a year of my transformation. Chapter 1 (year 1), was the year I had an epiphany. It was also the year that I had to finally come face to face with some disturbing behaviors and suppressed emotions I didn't want to recognize, but it was necessary for me to acknowledge, accept, change, and then move forward.

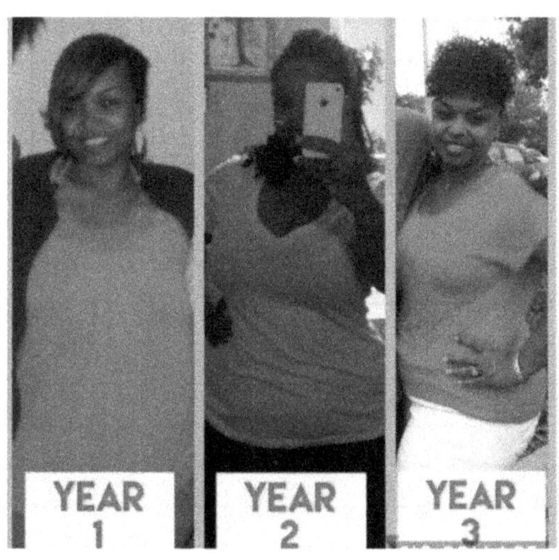

It was actually my birthday in the year 1 picture. I was 33 years old, and in the WORST physical shape of my life. At 180lbs, I constantly told myself that it "wasn't that bad", that I might as well just be "fat and happy", and I had convinced myself that I just *couldn't* lose the weight. Everything I had tried before failed, so why even waste my time again and face disappointment? The smile on my face is a fake one. I pretended to be so happy to be celebrating my birthday with friends, but the minute I was in my car, I felt lonely, depressed, and ashamed of how far gone I allowed myself to get. Yet despite the momentary pity party I was having, I still carried on as usual, eating the same way I always did and living a sedentary lifestyle. That is, until about a week or so later when my family and I ventured to Daytona Beach (and the morbid pizza shop window woke me up). I had finally made up my mind that enough was enough. I wasn't going to continue with the dumb excuses, and it was better for me to *fail forward*, then to not try at all! Yes, I failed. Numerous times I'd fall, cry, scream, give up, get angry, frustrated, anxious, worried, but I GOT BACK UP every day and tried again.

I'm probably the only person that will tell you with total transparency – in the beginning, middle, and continuation of your health journey; it's inevitable – YOU WILL FAIL. There is no such thing as getting everything right 100% all of the time. There will be many days when you will not want to work out. Days when you will want to say forget this crap and go for a large pizza instead of boring grilled chicken breast and broccoli. You'll have plenty of days when you'll flat out say "I'M DONE!", yet you'll muster up the strength to keep going.

Year 1 was the year of REALIZATION. I realized that I had several problems and I needed to do something about it. I wasn't comfortable in my own skin and I hated the way I looked and felt about myself. I also realized that I had the ability to change my situation. I realized my own strength. I realized that I could do anything if I actually made the effort to do the work. I learned very quickly that what I wanted to accomplished wouldn't take place in a few weeks, or a few months. It was going to be a process.

I originally set a goal to lose just 15lbs and to get back into a loose size 10 (that was the size I wore my entire adult life up until gaining the excess weight). As I started the process, I realized something else – I set the bar way too low. I wanted to not just lose 15 lbs., but I wanted to strive to become the best "me" I could be! Soon, 15lbs turned into wanting to lose 20 lbs., then it turned into a 25lb goal, and so on.

The more I learned about fitness, food, and overall health in general, the more addictive it became. Were there days I wanted to forget everything and go back to eating junk and not exercising? ABSOLUTELY. But it was on those days I had to go back and remember *why* I started the process in the first place. One thing that really kept me motivated was looking at my day 1 picture. All of the negative emotions I felt looking at the picture came flooding right back, and it pushed me to get up off my behind, or put down the crap I was getting ready to eat to get back to business!

Speaking of pictures – THEY WORK! You will feel like you've made zero progress when you look in the mirror (and remember scales don't tell the full truth), and that's because you look at yourself every day, so it's very hard to see where you've made any real changes. Taking pictures is a sure way to be able to track your progress and see big differences as you go through the process. Take a day 1 picture when you first begin (take front, back, and both sides), and every month thereafter take another picture and compare them to the last. You'll more than likely be amazed at the differences you'll see, even if the scale doesn't tell you!

As the months rolled by and I started noticing subtle changes, my confidence started to increase, I started making more conscience decisions regarding my eating habits, and I actually started to enjoy and look forward to exercising (me, the same woman who couldn't stand the thought of working out turned into an exercise junkie!). The next thing I knew, a full year had gone by and I had lost a TON of inches all over my body (I lost an entire FOOT off my waist – 12 inches! and was starting to see my hourglass curves again!).

Along with taking pictures, record your measurements! From day 1, measure every part of your body – arm width, thighs, hips, waist, chest/bust, ankles, everything! This is also a real way to measure your progress along with pictures. Overall for year 1, I had lost about 18 lbs. The weight doesn't seem like a lot to have lost in a full year, but considering the inches that was gone (all from fat loss – remember the scale doesn't tell you the real story!), I had dropped from a tight size 14 into a loose 9/10 by the time year 2 came around.

Year 2 definitely started off way better than the year before. I had settled into a routine, had adjusted to the different eating habits, and had become a fitness junkie! When I say "junkie", I mean that in every form of the word – buying every workout blue-ray or digital product I could get, buying all the cute workout clothes, sneakers, sports bras, etc., and let me not forget the extensive collection of heavy weights, belts, mats, gloves, and anything else I could find to help me on my journey. I still had those days when I just didn't want to exercise, and days when I wanted to venture off my clean eating habits, but even when I wavered (and you WILL waver, and that's ok!), I regrouped, refocused, and got right back on track.

I started seeing real changes happening; not just physical, but my self-esteem and self-worth had drastically increased. I went from not wearing dresses at all (because I couldn't stand my knees or the way dresses looked on me), to buying an entire wardrobe full of them. I actually started feeling good about myself, and at that point, I couldn't remember the last time I felt that way. I was in a comfortable size 10 (which was my original goal), but I decided to just keep going to get even more toned and healthier. I had lost around 25lbs total and a whopping 56 inches combined on all parts of my body. My body fat percentage had dropped by 15%.   I was so excited to finally be finding myself again! It's so easy to get lost in the everyday shuffle of being a wife, mother, employee, friend, aunt, sister, and the list goes on and on. I was so busy taking care of everyone else that I forgot about 'me'. This was the year I was truly starting to see the woman I knew was hiding under all of that excess weight for several years. But boy oh boy, when life happens, it happens with a vengeance and eventually I became complacent and comfortable. I found myself slipping back into old habits.

Year 3 I fell off the wagon in a big way. The stresses of a job I couldn't stand, being a fulltime wife and mother, dealing with illnesses, family members dying, and a host of other life events that took place totally threw me for a loop. It seemed like everything and everyone was keeping me from being able to refocus my efforts to staying in a healthy lifestyle. I started eating out again… A LOT. I started slipping back into barely working out 2-3 times a week when I was working out 5-6 times a week the year prior. I even stopped using the scale altogether as a tool to help me gauge my weight fluctuations. A full 6 months had gone by and I didn't get on the scale, didn't take any measurements, and was barely watching what I ate.

The truth of the matter was I knew I had messed up big time. I knew that I was hurting myself by falling back into sedentary habits. Even worse, I already knew that the scale was going to tell me just how horrible I had really been over the last 6 months. In my mind, I figured I had maybe gained only a few pounds back. I ignored the fact that my belly was starting to swell again and that my pants were getting tighter and tighter by the week.

So one Saturday I reluctantly decided to get on both my digital scale and spring scale. When I looked down at what I was facing, I could feel the blood rush from my face. I was terrified at the numbers that showed up. It had to be an error, right? I stared at the numbers that stared back at me and thought "this can't be possible"! I jumped from one scale to the next and both kept mocking me with similar results – I had gained back 23 of the 25lbs I had lost! Keeping in mind that my body type is Endomorph (it's incredibly easy for me to gain weight and store fat, but not so easy to come off), so just the thought of having to start from the bottom again petrified me.

U-N-B-E-L-I-E-V-A-B-L-E was the only thing I could think of at the time, before bursting into crocodile tears for literally hours. How could I allow that to happen? What was I thinking? How could I be so careless and stupid? How could I allow myself to basically go right back to square one? These were just a few questions I beat myself over the head with the entire day. Detriment, disgust, bewilderment, anguish, panic, disappointment, discouragement, and defeat were only a few of the emotions that ran through my mind. As horrible as it felt, it was a wakeup call for me to get my butt back in gear and get it together. I sucked it up, acknowledged my mistakes, put my big girl panties on, and got off the pity party train. The following day, I hit the reset button and went full speed ahead...

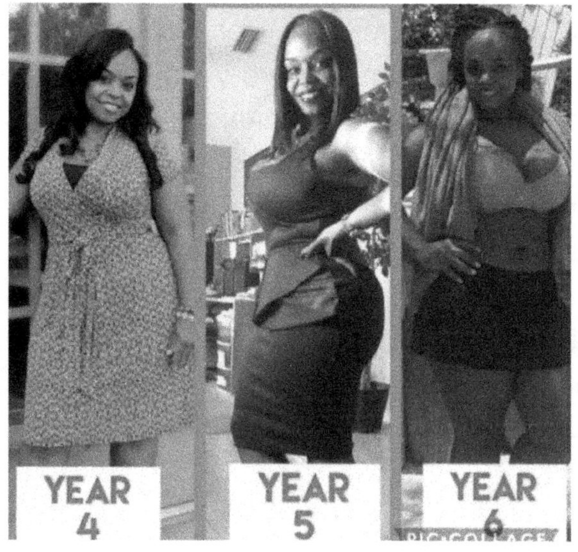

Year 4 was slightly challenging. After falling back into old habits, it was difficult to reprogram my thinking, but I knew it could be done. If I did it before, I could certainly do it again! I reminded myself that we all fall from time to time; but it's the getting back up that counts. The most valuable lesson I learned in that season was that mistakes happen, I'm not perfect, and it does me no good beating myself up for not staying committed. Bottom line – I didn't dwell on it and decided to pick up the pieces and move forward.

Slowly but surely, I found myself getting back into the "groove" of working out every day, drastically cut back on eating out, started drinking nothing but water again, and started refocusing my thinking back to the original purpose – to get healthy and stay healthy. After a few months, the weight started falling back off again, but this time because my body was already conditioned from the prior few years it was an easier process. That is, until I hit a major brick wall: the PLATEAU.

Understand that as you lose weight, your metabolism starts to slow down which causes your body to burn less calories than when you initially begin losing weight. The slower metabolism will slow down weight loss despite still eating lower calories and working out.[32] When this happens, your body has reached a "plateau" or has "leveled off". I would be lying if I said this part of the journey didn't frustrate the living daylights out of me. It's a real bummer to be working hard and eating right, only for the progress to be stalled, and there's no way around it. I just had to accept it (because it is what it is and

---

[32] Mayo Clinic Staff. 2015. "Getting Past the Weight Loss Plateau". https://www.mayoclinic.org/healthy-lifestyle/weight-loss/in-depth/weight-loss-plateau/art-20044615

being upset wasn't going to change it), so I made the slight adjustments required to break through it:

- **I reassessed my eating habits.** Was I eating too many bad carbs? Did I overeat? Did I miss too many meals (because that's not good either)?
- **I cut a few more calories.** I made sure to rev up my veggies and lean proteins, and cut back on the things I was allowing such a butter, breads, and anything else that I felt contributed to the slow down.
- **I increased my workout time.** I added more weight training into the mix, along with adding extra minutes to my cardio, or doing an extra workout or 2 per week. Weightlifting increases your muscle mass will help you burn more calories.
- **I added more activities throughout the day.** I parked far from stores and walked, I took the stairs whenever possible, etc.

Eventually, I overcame the plateau (and there has been more than 1 over the years), but the only way to get pass it is through persistence and perseverance.

Lesson: You simply can't give up when it gets "too hard".

Year 5 & Year 6 was what I would consider my break out years. I had even amazed myself with how far I had come and had surpassed my original goal of just losing "10-15lbs" and getting into a loose size 10. I reached a size 4/6 in dresses and a size 7/8 in pants – sizes I had never in my adult life had ever worn. Weight wise, I noticed it fluctuated between 145-155lbs based on drastically increasing my muscle mass, hormonal changes, water weight, and waste that hadn't been eliminated. It's so easy to get stuck on numbers and immediately become discouraged, but I had to keep reminding myself that I had come a mighty long way, that I was still very happy with my overall progress, I was happy with the size I was, and I finally was beginning to feel good in my own skin. Most importantly, I reminded myself that I would NEVER return to where I first began!

I increased weight training from year 5 to year 6, making me appear slightly thicker, but carrying more lean muscle. In present day, I have maintained the same weight range and continue to watch what I eat, and continue to work out at least 5 days a week. I fully understand my body and I know what works and what doesn't. Being that it's so hard for my body type to lose weight, I have to work extra hard at maintaining my progress.

It can be very annoying at times. There are many days when I want to just sit and eat several slices of supreme pizza and guzzle down an ice cold Pepsi®, but instead of eating several slices, I may have 1 slice (and split it in half so I can eat it slower – mind tricks!), and fill my plate up with salad with low calorie dressing instead, and still satisfy my craving without over indulging. I have become a serious water lover over the last few years, so honestly I can take or leave sodas and juices. I don't miss them at all, and can count how many times on 1 hand I drink anything other than water in a year. If I get a craving to have something other than plain water, I opt for extremely low calorie Crystal Light®, preferably fruit punch, which tastes more like cherry Kool-Aid®. It becomes easy to swap out old favorites with healthier versions and not lose the flavor.

In Chapter 6, you'll see several breakfast, lunch, dinner, snack and even dessert recipes that I personally use that are easy alternatives to the less healthy versions. I absolutely LOVE FOOD! But those nasty pre-made diet dinners and fake alternatives (fake cheese, meat, etc.), are not up my alley. I'm an old school cook and a custom baker so I'm a true foodie. There is no way I could maintain my healthy lifestyle by eating disgusting food. I've learned to make adjustments and still make food taste just as tasty as when they were filled with extra fats and preservatives.

Also, please understand that I definitely know how to LIVE as my son reminded me. I will go through a Krispy Kreme® drive-thru every blue moon when that dreaded "Hot Now" light comes on! I'll eat 1 super delicious donut that satisfies my craving, then give the rest to my kids and their friends to enjoy. Note I didn't say it was "easy" to only eat 1, but I was *disciplined* enough to stop at what I allowed myself to enjoy without guilt.

I also increase my water intake right after eating something "not so healthy" to flush my system faster. The magic word is MODERATION. You can still enjoy all that life has to offer within limits. Life is meant to be enjoyed, and it's also about what you make it. It's not meant to be all rules, restrictions, and a bunch of do's and don'ts.

I have learned throughout my journey (and it's a continuum), that I don't have to be a prisoner in my own body or mind. I have the ability to change what needs to be changed, and the ability to control what needs to be controlled. All I can do is give my best, and God will do the rest. You too, will get to the place where you've reached your goal, and will be able to look back and be proud of what you've achieved, and turn around and help someone else reach their goal! The fact that you are reading this book is living proof that ALL things are possible.

POINTS TO PONDER…

Your Journey is YOURS. Just like all of our body types are uniquely assigned to us through genetics, your journey is yours alone. You may not be able to control every aspect of the journey, but you can control your reaction!

Forget the "Quick Fixes". If you think reaching your goals will happen through some "quick fix", you're in for some great disappointment. Please note that my journey has been a process of over 6 years, and continues to this day. To get permanent and lasting results, it calls for a total CHANGE. I can't say that enough. You may lose a few pounds on a fad diet initially, but the weight will come back with a vengeance and add a few extra "friends" to go along with it.

Be PATIENT. If anyone understands how frustrating it is to wants something so badly and it seems to take forever to be achieved, it's me. Don't try to eat the entire elephant in one sitting; take it one piece at a time, one day at a time, and one week at a time and so on.

Set Realistic Goals. One of the biggest mistakes most people make when venturing into weight loss is setting unrealistic goals in the beginning. To say off the top that you want to lose 50lbs will seem like 500lbs when you haven't even reached 5lbs! Initially I set a goal of 10-15lbs, but even that seemed too grandiose. I broke it down into 5lb chunks to make it more achievable. The next thing I knew, I had surpassed those goals and had moved onto the next.

You may fall, but you can't stay there. GET BACK UP! Having a long drawn out pity party for messing up is only going to make matters worse. Get up, dust yourself off, reassess what you need to do to correct your mistakes and get back on the horse – quickly! The longer you allow yourself to stay down, the harder it will be to get back on track. Trust me, I speak from experience.

CHAPTER 5

TOP RECOMMENDED

"READS"

"True You: A Journey to Finding and Loving Yourself" by Janet Jackson and David Ritz

"Daily Word for Weight Loss: Spiritual Guidance to Give you Courage on Your Journey" by Colleen Zuck and Elaine Meyer

"Mini Habits for Weight Loss: Stop Dieting. Form New Habits. Change your Lifestyle without Suffering" By Stephen Guise

"The Truth about Beauty: Transform your Looks and your Life from the Inside Out" by Kat James and Oz Garcia

NOTES

Chapter 6:
Real Food, Real Results

No health journey is easy if you're eating cardboard for breakfast, lunch and dinner. I have certainly tried all the gross meal plans and meal "systems", and they left me discouraged and miserable. My thoughts were, "Was this really how I was going to have to eat to lose weight?" "Is this all I have to look forward to for the days, weeks, and years to come?" Food is one of life's pleasures that should always be doing 2 things:

1. **Food should provide sustenance to your body**. If it has a ton of gibberish scientific words in the ingredients, then it's more than liking poisoning you.

   Nutrients, vitamins, and medicinal properties should be provided through what we eat. It shouldn't be that artificial medications take the place of what God has already provided to grow, clean, and protect our bodies.

2. **Food should be Fun!** There is a difference between enjoying what you eat and overindulging. There is no rule that says you can't have fun with your food in how it's prepared (as long as you're mindful to stay away from greasy, fried, smothered, and butter slathered cooking methods), or the visual presentation of the food.

We eat with our eyes first, then with our mouth. Think of all the cooking shows you've seen and nice restaurants you've visited. Visual presentation is what makes food appeal to be enticing and tantalizing to the senses. Why not make your own food look and taste just as good?

In this day and age, everything has to be bigger, faster, and more convenient. For most of us, it's because of TIME (or lack thereof), lack of knowledge, and lack of convenience. There's no easy solution for either reason – you either make time for food prep or you don't. You either take the time to learn or re-learn how to cook or you don't. Last, you either learn how to slow down long enough to find new methods to make prepping food more convenient or you don't. It boils down to a matter of CHOICE.

For years I made up the excuse that I didn't have time to cook healthy food and I didn't have time to look up any new recipes (but I had time to scroll through social media and watch TV). When it comes to changing your health, it starts with what you put in your body! MAKE THE TIME! Do the work required. We make time to do what we *want* to do, and not what we *need* to do. Note that the title of this chapter says "*real food*". Real can't be substituted; it either is or it isn't.

It can be hard in the beginning to change your eating habits, but it helps if you focus on small changes. The first thing I did when making changes was cutting back on unhealthy fat. Unhealthy fats include: dark chicken meat (thighs and legs); chicken skin; fatty cuts of beef, pork, and lamb, and high-fat dairy foods (whole milk, butter, cheeses). If you currently eat a lot of fat, make a commitment to cutting back ASAP.

Here are some quick tips to help you make immediate changes:

- Instead of frying meat, try baking, grilling, or broiling it. Remove the skin from chicken and turkey because the skin is all fat.
- Drastically increase any extra fat. This includes full fat salad dressings, sour cream, mayonnaise, and butter. Opt for low fat or no-fat versions instead. One of my favorite salad dressings is 'Opa by Litehouse'®. It's miniscule in calories

because it's a Greek yogurt based dressing, but tastes delicious!

- Eat plenty of fruits and vegetables for snacks and with your meals.
- Drink zero- or low-calorie beverages, such as water or unsweetened tea. Sweetened drinks add lots of calories to your diet such as fruit juice, soda, sports drinks, coffee drinks, and sweet tea.
- When it comes to eating out, be sure to pack ½ your meal away at the beginning so you're not tempted to overeat. Restaurants give humongous portions. Also don't be afraid to ask for food to be prepared a certain way to fit your needs.

Its small steps like making subtle changes that lead to big results. There is so much that could be discussed about how food is grown, processed, developed, marketed, and contributes to current illnesses and deformities. There isn't enough time in the day to cover all of the gimmicks, tricks, chemicals, hormones, and other very harmful methods used in the food industry today, all for the sake of the mighty dollar.

The goal of this chapter isn't to drown you in a ton of dietary facts, but to provide some simple yet tasty recipes and ideas to help you jump start your healthy eating habits. Even if you don't like to cook or know how to cook, these recipes should be simple enough for you to follow to get you going in the right direction. The next few pages are broken into 5 categories: **Breakfast, Lunch, Dinner, Snacks,** and **Desserts.**

Each section will have a week's worth of sample recipes that will help you kick start changing your cooking regimen. All are recipes that I personally enjoy, but feel free to substitute different fruits, grains, etc. as long as they add up to the same calorie, sugar, and fat amounts as in the recipe.

Please note that if there is an ingredient that doesn't cater to your taste buds, or you have an ALLERGY against a certain food listed, find a healthy alternative to use in its place. Also, if you are vegetarian, opt to replace traditional meat for high protein meat substitutes such as tofu or tempeh.

Hopefully, you will get the same enjoyment from these delicious recipes[33] (some derived from

---

[33] "Healthy Ideas that will Promote Weight Loss". 2017. https://www.womenshealthmag.com/weight-loss/healthy-breakfast-ideas

Women's Health Magazine, and some from personal recipes) as I have over the years!

BREAKFAST

Breakfast is exactly as the name implies: Break-Fast. When you eat in the morning after sleeping, you're literally breaking the fast your body has been on since you went to sleep. Starting your day off with the right proteins and nutrients can set the stage for the rest of your day, giving you the energy you need.

EGG QUESADILLA
1 whole egg plus 1 egg white
2 Tbsp chopped green pepper
2 Tbsp chopped red onion
1 8-inch whole-wheat tortilla
1 oz Monterey Jack cheese, shredded
2 Tbsp chunky salsa

Scramble eggs with pepper and onion, and fold into tortilla with cheese and salsa.

Total: *330 calories*

This meal carries 20 grams of protein, which is essential in losing weight.

OATMEAL WITH PECANS AND BERRIES

1 packet Original Quaker Instant Oatmeal
1 cup skim milk
2 Tbsp chopped pecans
1/2 cup raspberries
1/2 cup blueberries

Use milk to prepare oatmeal according to package directions, and mix in pecans, raspberries, and blueberries.

Total: *351 calories*

Oatmeal is full of fiber and will keep you full much longer than the average grain.

TROPICAL YOGURT WITH CINNAMON TOAST

6 oz Fage Total 0% Greek Yogurt
1/4 tsp coconut extract
6 pieces dried mango
2 slices cinnamon-raisin bread

Mix coconut extract into yogurt, and sprinkle chopped mango on top. Enjoy cinnamon-raisin bread toasted.
Total: *394 calories*

BREAKFAST BURRITO

2 egg whites
2 whole-wheat tortillas
1/4 cup fat-free cheese
1/4 cup rinsed black beans
Salsa

Scramble the egg whites to desired degree of doneness, then load onto tortillas along with cheese and beans. Roll up, microwave for 30 seconds, and top with salsa.

Total: *282 calories*

BERRY BREAKFAST SMOOTHIE

1 banana, cut into chunks
1/2 cup nonfat milk
1/4 cup frozen unsweetened blueberries
1/4 cup frozen unsweetened strawberries
1 tsp peanut butter
1/2 tsp honey

In a blender, combine the banana, milk, blueberries, strawberries, peanut butter, and honey. Process about 1 minute, or until the consistency of a thick milkshake.

Total: *225 calories*

FRENCH TOAST WITH STRAWBERRIES
1 egg
2 Tbsp nonfat milk
2 slices whole-wheat bread
13 strawberries, sliced
1/2 tsp powdered sugar

Whisk together egg and milk, and dip bread into mixture. Cook in nonstick pan until slightly browned. Top with berries and sugar.

Total: *275 calories*

Strawberries are powerful little fruits. The fiber in them helps alleviate hunger and also helps ward off breast cancer and diabetes.

EGG-WHITE FRITTATA WITH FETA, SPINACH, AND MUSHROOMS
2 egg whites
1 egg
1/2 cup chopped fresh spinach
1/2 cup chopped button mushrooms
1 oz feta cheese

1 tsp fresh cilantro
1 slice oat-bran bread

Whisk together the egg and egg whites. In a skillet misted with cooking spray, cook mushrooms and spinach over medium heat until spinach is wilted. Reduce to low heat, and add eggs. Cover, and cook 3 minutes, until eggs are firm. Top with feta and cilantro. Serve with toast.

Total: *362 calories*

If necessary for the sake of allergies, feel free to use alternatives to peanut butter, eggs, cheeses, etc. that fit your dietary needs.

LUNCH

Since lunch in midday, you'll should eat something that's filling but not going to make you drowsy like the results of eating an extremely heavy meal. It also helps that these recipes are quick and easy to prep.

TACO SALAD
4 oz ground turkey (93% lean)
1 1/2 tsp Simply Organic Southwest Taco seasoning
3 cups shredded romaine lettuce
1/4 cup black beans
1/2 cup diced tomatoes

1/4 cup yellow corn
1 Tbsp Mexican or Taco Blend cheese
5 blue-corn tortilla chips, crumbled (if desired)

Brown turkey in a pan on the stove top, and stir in taco seasoning. Toss turkey with remaining ingredients.

Total: *410 calories*

CHICKEN PANINI

1 1/2 oz sliced low-fat Swiss
1 oz sliced reduced-sodium Black Forest deli ham
1 oz sliced reduced-sodium deli chicken breast
1 whole-wheat roll (12 oz total), sliced and <u>gutted</u>
1/4 cup marinara sauce, heated

Heat lightly oiled grill or Panini press to medium heat (or use a grill pan). Place cheese, ham, and chicken on the roll, starting and ending with cheese. Close sandwich, and grill, flipping and pressing with spatula if necessary, until golden brown on both sides and cheese is melted, about five minutes total. Halve sandwich, and serve with marinara sauce for dipping.

Total: *292 calories*

MOZZARELLA AND TOMATO SALAD
1 medium tomato, cubed
1 oz fresh part-skim mozzarella cheese, cubed
1 cup fresh spinach leaves
1 clove garlic, pressed
1 1/2 tsp olive oil
2 tbsp balsamic vinegar
1/4 tsp black pepper

Combine, and toss all ingredients.

Total: *243 calories*

Fresh Mozzarella is low in sodium and high in calcium and protein.

BBQ TURKEY BURGERS
1 pound ground dark-meat turkey
1 garlic clove, minced
1/2 teaspoon paprika
1/4 teaspoon ground cumin
Pinch of kosher salt
1/4 teaspoon freshly ground black pepper
4 slices sweet onion, grilled
1/4 cup barbecue sauce
4 (1.6-oz) sesame seed buns, toasted

In medium bowl, gently mix together turkey, garlic, paprika, and cumin. Form turkey into 4 (4-inch) patties; season with salt and pepper. Heat grill to medium-high; cook, turning once, until burgers are just cooked through (about 7 minutes per side). Serve with desired toppings and buns.

ROAST BEEF AND HORSERADISH WRAP

2 Tbsp 2% plain Greek yogurt
1 Tbsp horseradish sauce
2 leaves Bibb lettuce
4 slices lean deli-style roast beef
4 slices tomato
1 cup fresh berries (blueberries, raspberries, strawberries or mixed)

Combine the yogurt and horseradish, and spread on lettuce. Top with roast beef and tomato, and roll into a wrap. Serve with berries.

Total: *300 calories*

DIJON CHICKEN SALAD
1 cup roasted skinless chicken breast, cubed
1 Tbsp fresh lemon juice
4 tsp Dijon mustard
1/2 jalapeno, diced
1/2 medium celery stalk, chopped

Dash of black pepper
1 cup baby spinach

Combine the first six ingredients, and serve on a bed of spinach.

Total: *266 calories*

OPEN-FACED TURKEY AND FETA SANDWICH

1 slice whole-grain bread
3 oz sliced turkey breast
1/4 cup baby spinach
1/4 cup sun-dried tomatoes
1 Tbsp feta

Side Salad
12 yellow or red cherry tomatoes, halved
1/4 cup chopped cucumber
4 large black olives, chopped
1 Tbsp chopped scallion
1/2 Tbsp olive oil
1/2 tsp fresh lemon juice
1 tsp fresh mint

Top bread with turkey, spinach, sun-dried tomatoes, and feta. Broil six to eight minutes, or until golden. Serve with salad. **Total:** *367 calories*

DINNER

Dinner should be your lightest meal of the day, particularly because it's closer to you going to bed. Lighter doesn't mean it has to be boring or tasteless. The following are a few delicious ideas, all less than 500 calories!

HOT DOG W/BAKED BEANS

1 organic beef hot dog
1/2 cup organic baked beans
1 whole-wheat hot dog bun
1/2 Tbsp whole-grain mustard
1/2 Tbsp sweet relish
1 cup sliced watermelon

Cook hot dog, and heat baked beans in a saucepan. Serve hot dog in the bun, topped with mustard and relish, with beans and melon on the side.

Total: *490 calories*

Be sure to NOT load your hotdog with anything other than mustard and/or relish to keep calories low.

QUICK CHICKEN SOUP WITH ASPARAGUS

4 oz boneless, skinless chicken breast
1 cup Organic Chunky Vegetable soup
2 Tbsp dry quinoa
1 cup chopped kale
10 small asparagus spears
2 tsp soy sauce
1/8 tsp grated fresh ginger

Bake chicken at 350°F for 25 minutes, then shred with a fork. Meanwhile, combine soup, quinoa, and kale in a saucepan, bring to a boil, and simmer until quinoa is done, about 15 minutes. Add chicken. Steam asparagus, then toss with soy sauce and ginger. Serve asparagus on the side.

TOTAL: *330 calories*

PORK TENDERLOIN WITH VEGGIES

1 pork tenderloin (4 oz)
1 cup steamed green beans
2 Tbsp sliced almonds
1 baked sweet potato

Season pork with salt and pepper, sear in an ovenproof skillet coated with cooking spray, and transfer to a 450°F oven for 15 minutes. Slice and serve with green beans topped with almonds, and a sweet potato.

Total: *370 calories*

Although I typically stay away from pork, tenderloin is an occasional exception because it is white meat that's high in protein and low in saturated fat.

BAKED CHICKEN WITH MUSHROOMS AND SWEET POTATO

1/2 skinless chicken breast
1 cup baby portobello mushrooms, sliced
1 Tbsp chives
1 Tbsp olive oil
1 medium sweet potato

In a 350°F oven, bake chicken, topped with mushrooms, chives, and oil, for 15 minutes. Microwave sweet potato for five to seven minutes.

Total: *382 calories*

CHICKEN PESTO PASTA

1/4 pint cherry tomatoes
1/3 cup cooked green beans
1/3 cup diced chicken breast
1/4 cup pesto sauce
1/4 tsp each salt and pepper
1 cup cooked linguine
1/4 cup shredded Parmesan

Combine tomatoes, cooked green beans, diced chicken breast, pesto sauce, and salt and pepper in a bowl. Add cooked linguine. Garnish with shredded Parmesan.

Total: *417 calories*

ASIAN LETTUCE CUPS
4 oz ground lean turkey
1/2 cup white mushrooms, chopped
1 tsp minced garlic
1/4 cup shelled and cooked edamame
2 Boston lettuce leaves
2 Tbsp sliced scallion

Sauce
1/2 Tbsp hoisin sauce
1 tsp low-sodium soy sauce
1/2 tsp rice vinegar

Asian Slaw
1/2 cup shredded red cabbage and green cabbage
1/4 cup sliced jicama
1/4 cup grated carrot
1 tsp olive oil
1/2 tsp rice vinegar

In a nonstick skillet coated with cooking spray, sauté first three ingredients for five minutes. Add edamame, scoop mix onto lettuce, top with scallion, and wrap up. Drizzle with sauce, and serve slaw on the side.

Total: *329 calories*

TERIYAKI BEEF STIRFRY

3 oz grass-fed beef tenderloin, cubed
2 Tbsp reduced-sodium teriyaki sauce
1 Tbsp light honey-mustard dressing
2 tsp olive oil
1/4 cup sliced carrots
1/2 cup chopped broccoli
1/4 cup sliced water chestnuts
1/4 cup sliced peppers
1/2 cup cooked brown rice

Marinate beef in teriyaki and dressing for 30 minutes. Heat olive oil in a pan, and cook beef one to two minutes. Add veggies, and cook for another five to seven minutes until beef is browned. Serve over rice.

Total: *500 calories*

SNACKS

This is certainly not a comprehensive list of healthy snacks, but just a few out of hundreds of snack combinations you can create to curb your appetite. Whether you're craving something salty, crunchy, sweet, or savory, you should find something that would benefit you both in craving and in health benefits.

You should be eating 5-6 small meals a day (your 3 main meals with snacks in between, or all mini meals). Having a healthy snack in between meals is a sure way to keep from overindulging when you do eat, keeps your blood sugar level, and staves off hunger which leads to poor snack choices. Here are some great healthy snack options to try:

- Pouched Fish (Tuna, Salmon)
- Hard-Boiled Eggs (1-2)
- Turkey breast rollup w/Swiss cheese (1)
- Sunflower seeds (unsalted, ½ cup)
- Pickle (1)
- 5 Shrimp w/cocktail sauce
- Sugar-free Jell-O (1 cup)
- Frozen Yogurt (1 cup max)
- Protein Bars (1)
- Apple (1 medium)

- Orange (1 medium)
- Banana
- Plain Greek Yogurt (1 cup)
- String Cheese (1)
- Peanut Butter (1 TBSP)
- Almond Butter (1 TSBP)
- Air Popped Popcorn (2 cups)
- Mixed Nuts (a handful, as they can also be high in fat)
- Frozen Grapes (1 cup)
- Strawberries (1 cup) Try them as "strawberries and cream" with 1-2 TBSP Sugar Free Cool Whip ®.
- Kale Chips (liberty)
- Dark Chocolate (1-2oz)
- Unsweetened Applesauce (1/2 cup)
- Laughing Cow® cheese (1 wedge with 3-4 whole wheat crackers)
- Hummus & veggies (1/2 cup)
- Guacamole & Veggies (1/2 cup)
- Green tea (1 cup)
- Black Coffee (1 cup)
- Low calorie Fruit and/or Veggie Smoothies (6-8oz)
- Apples slices with peanut butter (1 medium apple and 1 TBSP peanut butter)

High-Protein Banana and Peanut Butter

Mix half a tablespoon of peanut butter with half an ounce of protein powder and half an ounce of water. Cut half a banana in half lengthwise. Smear the peanut butter mixture on half and then top with the other half of the banana.

Skinny Crab-Deviled Eggs

4 large hard-boiled eggs
4 tsp mayonnaise
1 tsp Dijon mustard
1 Tbsp. chopped green onions
¼ c lump crabmeat, shells removed

1. **CUT** the eggs lengthwise.
2. **REMOVE** the yolks and place them in a mixing bowl.
3. **MASH** with a fork and stir in the mayonnaise and mustard.
4. **FOLD** in the green onion.
5. **SPOON** about a tablespoon of the mixture into each egg white half and top with the crab-meat. **52 Calories each**

Homemade Granola Bars

2 c old-fashioned rolled oats
¼ c ground flaxseed
¾ tsp ground cinnamon
¼ tsp ground cloves
¼ tsp salt
½ c almond butter
¼ c honey
1 tsp vanilla extract
½ c finely chopped and pitted dates or raisins
½ c dried cherries or goji berries

1. PREHEAT the oven to 350°F. Coat an 8" x 8" pan with canola oil cooking spray.
2. COMBINE the oats, flaxseed meal, cinnamon, cloves, and salt in a large bowl.
3. COMBINE the almond butter, honey, and vanilla in a small bowl. Add to the dry ingredients and stir to combine. Stir in the dates and cherries until well combined.
4. PRESS the mixture firmly into the prepared pan.
5. BAKE for 25 minutes, or until the edges are browned. Let it cool completely before cutting into eight bars.
6. STORE in an airtight container.

 276 Calories per bar

Yogurt Dip and Veggies

32 oz fat-free plain yogurt
Garlic powder to taste
Onion powder to taste
Seasoned salt to taste
Cut-up fresh veggies

1. LINE a strainer with a coffee filter or white paper towel. Place the strainer over a bowl (this catches the liquid that will drain off the yogurt). Spoon the yogurt into the filter-lined strainer.
2. COVER and refrigerate for 8 hours or overnight. This process yields about 16 ounces of yogurt cheese.
3. SEASON the cheese lightly with the seasonings suggested above, or add freshly chopped herbs such as parsley, rosemary or thyme. Use as dip for fresh vegetables. **34 calories per ¼ cup**

DESSERT

Yes! Although you may be venturing into a healthy lifestyle, it doesn't mean you have to hang your love of sweets up completely. Being that I am the owner of a custom bakery, and a dessert lover to the bone, I have experience with creating baked and non-baked dessert methods that satisfies my sweet tooth, but doesn't affect my progress or my waistline. No you can truly have your dessert and eat it too!

Greek Yogurt Parfait
3/4 cup fat-free plain Greek yogurt
2 cups sliced fruit (whatever your favorite is! I use blueberries and strawberries)
3/4 cup puffed rice cereal
2 tablespoons walnuts and almonds, toasted and chopped
1 tablespoon ground flaxseed
1 tablespoon maple syrup, agave nectar, or honey

In a tall 4-cup container or jar, layer half of the yogurt, fruit, cereal, nuts, flaxseed, and syrup. Repeat with the remaining half of ingredients, ending with syrup. (If you prefer a crunchy parfait, pack cereal separately to add right before eating.) Refrigerate up to 5 hours.

Chocolate Dipped Bananas
2 tablespoons semisweet chocolate chips
1 small banana, peeled and cut into 1-inch chunks

Place chocolate chips in a heavy-duty zip-top plastic bag or small microwave-safe bowl.

Microwave at HIGH 1 minute or until chocolate melts. Dip banana pieces in chocolate and freeze until chocolate is firm.

*Alternative: Banana Pops – Leave banana whole and insert a popsicle stick half way up, then dip into chocolate coating under covered and freeze.

Chocolate Mousse-Filled Strawberries
1 can coconut milk
1/4 cup unsweetened cocoa powder
1/2 teaspoon vanilla extract
Sweetener to taste (Splenda, agave nectar, or honey)
Dash of salt
10-12 Strawberries (more if the mousse stretches)
Chopped almonds

Put coconut milk in the freezer for 20 minutes or leave it in the fridge overnight. The coconut milk should separate into half a watery mixture and half a white solid. Remove can from freezer or refrigerator and turn it upside down, open the bottom with a can opener, and pour out the watery liquid on top. There should be the white solid coconut milk at the bottom.

Combine coconut milk solid, cocoa power, vanilla extract, and salt in a mixer and blend until completely combined. Use a small knife to hollow out the center of each strawberry. Fill a sandwich bag with the mousse, and snip one of the corners so you can pipe the mousse into the strawberries. Finely chop some almonds (or whatever kind of nuts you want) and roll the tops of the filled strawberries in the chopped nuts. . Let the mixture chill for about 20 minutes in the fridge. Guilt-free treats to enjoy!

Healthy Peanut Butter Cookies
1 cup natural, smooth organic peanut butter (it should be smooth and drippy)

1/2 cup coconut sugar (can be found in The Fresh Market, Earth Fare, Whole Foods, and other stores that sell alternative ingredients)
1 large organic egg

Preheat oven to 350 degrees F.
Combine all ingredients in a large bowl.
Line a baking sheet with parchment or a silicone mat.
Roll dough into 12 balls and flatten lightly with the palm of your hand.
Using a fork, score cookies in opposite directions while flatten slightly more.
Bake for 12 minutes.

Remove cookies from oven and let sit on baking sheet for at least 10 minutes before removing and either serving or storing.

Churro Cheesecake Dip
1 (8 oz.) package Fat-free or light cream cheese, softened
3 tbsp. butter, softened
3 packets Splenda® OR 1 TBSP organic honey
½ tsp. vanilla extract
2 tsp. cinnamon
1/8 tsp. salt
1 apple, sliced for dipping

In a large bowl, beat light cream cheese and butter until light and fluffy. Add SPLENDA® Naturals Stevia Sweetener, vanilla, cinnamon, and salt and beat until incorporated. Serve with sliced green apples.

Apple Nachos
4 Granny Smith apples, sliced in wedges
1 c. white chocolate chips, melted
¾ c. sugar free caramel
1 c. chopped pretzels
½ c. Toffee Crunch (Heath brand found in chocolate chip section)

On a large plate, arrange apple slices on top of one another. Drizzle half the white chocolate and caramel, then top with pretzels and toffee crumbles. Drizzle with remaining white chocolate and caramel. Serve immediately.

Skinny Brownie Batter Dip
1 box Brownie Mix, Dry
2 c. fat free PLAIN yogurt
2 c. fat free or lite Cool Whip, thawed
½ c. mini chocolate chips

Combine brownie mix, yogurt, cool whip, and half the chocolate chips together in a large bowl until completely combined. Garnish with remaining chocolate chips and chill for 1 hour before serving. Great dippers: Fat free Vanilla wafers, Strawberries, Apples, Low-fat Graham crackers.

Remember, food should be pleasurable, not a burden. Eat all the foods you enjoy—but the key is to do it in smaller quantities and in moderation. The worst thing you can do is be too strict, then rebound by overeating all of the wrong things.

I have learned on my own journey that if you think of eating as something enjoyable and something you do without guilt and condemnation, as long as you stay very active, you'll be less likely to overeat and go astray from your goals. Make small changes to your eating habits one step, one day, one month at a time so you're not totally overwhelmed. Pretty soon, you'll be well on your way to be eating totally different and won't miss your old way of eating.

CHAPTER 6
TOP RECOMMENDED
"READS"

"The Healthy Meal Prep Cookbook: Easy and Wholesome Meals to Cook, Prep, Grab and Go" by Toby Amidor

"The Skinnytaste Cookbook: Light on Calories, Big on Flavor" by Gina Homolka

"The Laura Lea Balanced Cookbook: 120+ Everyday Recipes for the Healthy Home Cook" by Laura Lea and Alice Randall

"The Dude Diet: Clean(ish) Food for People Who like to Eat Dirty" by Serena Wolf

"Chocolate Covered Katie: Over 80 Delicious Recipes that are Secretly Good for You" by Katie Higgins

<u>Conclusion: And the Journey Begins…</u>

Welcome to the end and the beginning of your journey. By this point, it is my hope that you have been inspired, encouraged, empowered, and enlightened by my transparency with my ups and downs, my highs and my absolute lows.

It's typical to get to the end and forget major points as your processing all of the information. Here are some FINAL "Points to Ponder" for you to carry with you as you go forth and become the best YOU possible:

Chapter 1 – The Three "D's"

- **Dysmorphia and Depression** are both real mental illnesses that shouldn't be taken lightly. If you need to seek professional guidance, <u>please don't be ashamed or embarrassed to ask for the help</u> you need to feel better.

- **When it comes to diets**, learn how to create a permanent change instead of falling for all the diet fads and gimmicks that will more than likely leave you fatter, more frustrated and broke (diets aren't cheap!). Focus more on nourishment and what your body needs, not so much on rules and restrictions.

Chapter 2 - Numbers

- **Numbers take up a massive part of our world** and it's impossible to live without them. Although we need numbers, unhealthy obsessions with numbers can be crippling and stick you in a numerical prison.

- **Scales are only ONE part of the equation** to weight loss, only to be used as a tool and not as the full gospel truth about what's going on with your body.

- **Your worth is not dictated by the number** in your clothes! Be mindful of industry tricks of the trade to make you feel either skinnier or fatter to ploy you into buying.

Chapter 3 - The "F" Word

- **Regardless if you're having issues with Fitness, Food or Frustration,** there is never a "right time" to start eating the right food, there is never going to be a "perfect time" to start your fitness routine, and there will certainly never be a time when you won't have to face frustration. Just do the BEST you can do, and keep moving forward.

- **You have total dominion over your thoughts and your actions.** Just because a negative thought pops into your head doesn't mean you have to sign for it. Mentally stamp "return to sender" to the bad thoughts. ***Shut them down*** before they lead to other "stinkin' thinkin". Make a commitment today to start implementing actions that will make the "next" you, better than your "now" you!

Chapter 4 – Body Talk

- **Regardless** of how thin, thick, short, or tall you are, <u>everything about you is amazing</u>! You are not a mistake.

- **Stop comparing yourself** to someone who's had $10,000 worth of cosmetic surgery enhancements. Propaganda will coerce you into believing that are unrealistic, plastic, and airbrushed bodies are the ideal images of the "perfect body". Don't believe the hype!

- **Focus on what really matters** – fat loss. Instead of just focusing on what the scale or what a bias weight chart states, focus on your overall health and wellness.

Chapter 5 - The Journey

- **Accept your body for what it is,** then work towards making it a better version. Our body types are uniquely assigned to us through genetics, so there is no need to focus on the things you can't control. Work with the hand you were dealt from a positive place.

- **Change will NOT happen overnight.** If you think reaching your goals will happen through some "quick fix", you're sadly mistaken. You may lose a few pounds on a fad diet initially, but the weight typically returns and then some.

- **Set Realistic Goals.** One of the biggest mistakes most people make when venturing into weight loss is setting unrealistic goals. You may fall, but you can't stay there. GET BACK UP! Reassess what you need to do to correct your mistakes and quickly get back to work

Chapter 6: Real Food, Real Results

- **You can still eat and enjoy your food without overindulging.** You don't have to just eat lettuce for the rest of your life. What you eat accounts for about 80% of your weight loss (or gain) journey. The old saying is accurate – you ARE what you eat! A lifestyle change involves learning new methods of cooking that are better for your overall health, yet still retains tasty and enjoyable.

- **Make your journey an adventure!** Buy some new cookbooks, look up some cool recipes online, and try new foods that you ever thought you'd eat. Make the process an adventure. Learn about new spices and new ways of cooking your favorite dishes. You might just discover something amazing that you otherwise probably wouldn't have ever tried. Be open and receptive to learning and trying new foods.

It's my prayer that you have received something from this book that will help you become a better version of you. If you've gathered just 1 tip to use that you've never considered before, then I'd consider the purpose of this project a success. Your life is truly what you make it. One thing I have learned is that you can't start living when you feel like you've reached your goal weight, you have to start living RIGHT NOW.

In the illustrious words of the character Ellie Fredricksen from one of my favorite animated movies "UP", tell your old self, ***"Thanks for the Adventure – now go have a new one!"*** It's not a sprint, it's a JOURNEY. Enjoy it to the fullest!

<u>Works Cited</u>

(Numerical order)

[1] Philippians 4:13. 2015. New Living Translation Holy Bible.

2 Mark 11:23 New Living Translation, Holy Bible

[3] Merriam-Webster Learners Dictionary. 2016. "Wait".   http://www.merriam-webster.com/dictionary/wait

[4] Merriam-Webster Learners Dictionary. 2016. "Weight". http://www.merriam-webster.com/dictionary/weight

[5] Reference.com. 2016. *"How Much Time do we Spend   Waiting?"* *https://www.reference.com/science/much-time-spend-waiting-lifetime-2b089985e5384e65?qo=contentSimilarQuestions#*

6 Body Dysmorphic Disorder. Web MD 2016. http://www.webmd.com/mental-health/mental-health-body-dysmorphic-disorder

7 Body Dysmorphic Disorder. Written by Mayo Clinic Staff. Mayo Clinic 2016. http://www.mayoclinic.org/diseases-conditions/body-dysmorphic-disorder/symptoms-causes/dxc-20200938

[8] Adult Obesity Facts. 2015. Center for Disease Control & Prevention. http://www.cdc.gov/obesity/data/adult.html

[9] The Institute for the Psychology of Eating. 2016. *"3 Reasons Why Diets Don't Work." http://psychologyofeating.com/3-reasons-diets-dont-work/*

[10] The Institute for the Psychology of Eating. 2016. *"3 Reasons Why Diets Don't Work." http://psychologyofeating.com/3-reasons-diets-dont-work/*

[11] The Hormone Health Network. 2017. *"What Does Cortisol Do?"* http://www.hormone.org/hormones-and-health/what-do-hormones-do/cortisol

[12] Geary, Kevin. 2016. Rebooted Body 2016. "Why Diets Don't Work". http://rebootedbody.com/why-diets-dont-work/

13 Mayo Clinic Staff. 2016. "Metabolism & Weight Loss: How you burn Calories".

http://www.mayoclinic.org/healthy-lifestyle/weight-loss/in-depth/metabolism/art-20046508

[14] Poretsky, Golda, H.H.C. May 7 2012. "How to Break up with Dieting in 5 Easy Steps". http://www.bodylovewellness.com/2012/05/07/how-to-breakup-with-dieting-in-5-easy-steps/

[15] Hullett, Joseph, MD. August 3rd 2012. Major Depression Resource Center. "Weight loss Management for People with Depression". http://www.everydayhealth.com/hs/major-depression/weight-management-for-depression/

[16] Amen, Daniel G. MD. April 2nd 2013. "The Sane Way to Beat Anxiety and Depression". http://www.doctoroz.com/article/sane-way-beat-anxiety-and-depression?page=1

[17] Mayo Clinic Staff. 2016. "Depression: Major Depressive Disorder". http://www.mayoclinic.org/diseases-conditions/depression/in-depth/depression-and-exercise/art-20046495

[18] Scale (n). Merriam-Webster.com 2016. http://www.merriam-webster.com/dictionary/scale

[19] Faye, Denis M.S. July 21 2014. "4 Reasons working out can cause Weight Gain." Beach Body. http://www.beachbody.com/beachbodyblog/fitness/ask-the-expert-why-do-you-gain-weight-when-you-start-working-out

[20] Fitday. 2016. "The Four Best Types of Scales to Purchase". http://www.fitday.com/fitness-articles/fitness/weight-loss/the-four-best-types-of-scales-to-purchase.html

[21] Dockterman, Eliana. 2016. "Inside the fight to take back the fitting room". http://time.com/how-to-fix-vanity-sizing/

22 Triffin, Molly. November 12, 2010. "Vanity Sizing: The Insanity of size 0". http://www.cosmopolitan.com/style-beauty/fashion/advice/a3031/vanity-sizing/

[23] Zelman, Katherine M., MPH, RD, LD. WebMD 2005. Diet & Weight Management. "Estimated Calorie Requirements". http://www.webmd.com/diet/features/estimated-calorie-requirement

[24] Szalay, Jessie. 13 November 2015. Live Science. "What Are Calories?" http://www.livescience.com/52802-what-is-a-calorie.html

[25] Nichols, Lily RDN, CDE, CLT. 2014. "6 Reasons to Stop Counting Calories". http://pilatesnutritionist.com/6-reasons-to-stop-counting-calories-11-things-to-do-instead/

[26]Psalm 139:14. The Holy Bible. 2017. New Living Translation. BibleHub.com http://biblehub.com/psalms/139-14.htm

[27]Gomez, Alexandria. 1 August 2016. Women's Health. "Is Weight Loss really 80 Percent Diet and 20 percent Exercise?" http://www.womenshealthmag.com/weight-loss/weight-loss-80-percent-diet-20-percent-exercise

[28] Michi's Ladder. 2017. https://www.beachbodyondemand.com/blog/nutrition

[29]Spector, Dina. 14 May 2014. "How many days can a person survive without water". Science Business Insider. http://www.businessinsider.com/how-many-days-can-you-survive-without-water-2014-5

[30] "The 3 Body Types Explained: Ectomorph, Endomorph & Mesomorph". Taken 04 December 2017. http://www.directlyfitness.com/store/3-body-types-explained-ectomorph-mesomorph-endomorph/

[31] Johnson, John and Krista. 2017. "All these woman weight the same". Fit By Faith. http://www.fitbyfaith.net/motivational.html

[32] Photo credit: https://2weekstohealth.com/2017/04/26/the-difference-between-being-fat-and-overweight/

[33] Image Credit: "Fat vs. Muscle" Pinterest. 2017.

[34] "Healthy Ideas that will Promote Weight Loss". 2017. https://www.womenshealthmag.com/weight-loss/healthy-breakfast-ideas

About the Author

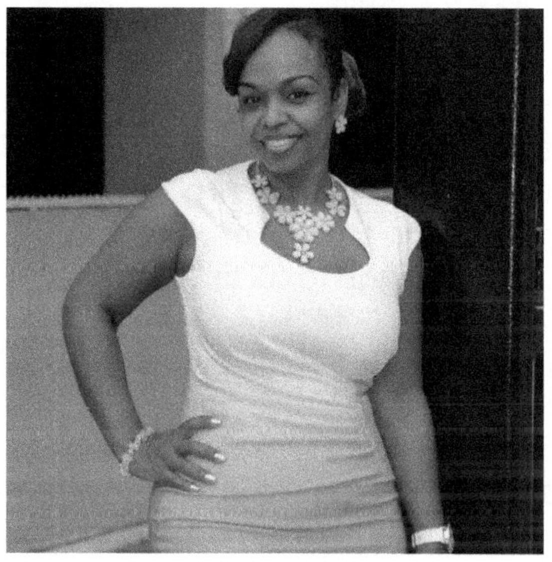

Juanita Jones is an established author, entrepreneur, motivational speaker and a woman with driven vision and in pursuit of fulfilling her purpose – to strengthen, encourage, and motivate others to walk out *their* purpose by Faith and to become their very BEST through the avenues of her business ventures.

She is the owner of Edible Blessings, LLC Custom Cakes and Desserts, specializing in custom desserts and exceptional services for all occasions. Her motto is, *"desserts should not only LOOK good, but actual TASTE as good as they look!"* Although Juanita established the business in 2002, she took a massive leap of faith in 2016 by leaving a lengthy career in Corporate Sales and Marketing to take her dream of Edible Blessings to fulltime status.

Aside from running a fulltime small business, in 2015, Juanita published her first book, "The Frustrated Dreamer: When your Dreams and Bigger than Your Now" – a book that combines raw, uncut truths regarding how to identify your purpose, how to recognize your "why", and how to execute your dreams in spite of how your current situation looks and feels.

As a result, she has appeared on local television talk shows, and has been a featured key note speaker for numerous non-profit organizations, schools, universities, conferences, and churches.

Juanita has a massive compassion for community services that benefit the infirmed, the poor, disadvantaged children, and for women battling emotional and mental issues. She is a natural giver at heart with her talent, time and treasure for numerous non-profit organizations, including:
Impact Church of Jacksonville, where she lends her writing/editing/proofing skills to the ministry;
Icing Smiles, Inc. – a nonprofit organization with a volunteer network of professional and novice bakers, who lend their talent for the creation of a custom "dream" cake for a mentally or physically ill child.

She also donates a portion of all sales from her books and from Edible Blessings, LLC to help those in need of food, clothing, utility bill assistance, transportation, educational needs, and any other need she sees fit to assist.

Juanita is an honor graduate from Park University with a BS degree in both Business Management and Human Resources, and currently has over 20+ years of sales, marketing, corporate training, public speaking, and business management experience.

Despite the numerous hats she wears and the rolls she plays, she believes that her greatest accomplishment is her family. She currently resides in Jacksonville, FL with her husband Steve, and their two sons, Jalil and Jalen.

FOLLOW JUANITA ON SOCIAL MEDIA

  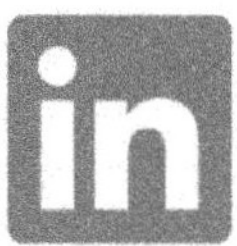

Dreamer Publications:
facebook.com/thefrustrateddreamer
(Follow here for more "AWEIGHTED" news!)

**Edible Blessings, LLC Custom Cakes &
Desserts:** facebook.com/edibleblessings
Instagram.com/edibleblessings
www.edibleblessin.com

LinkedIn:
linkedin.com/in/juanita-jones-2ab7b161/

To book for Speaking Engagements, Conferences, or other special events, please contact:
thefrustrateddreamer@hotmail.com

9 781982 042950